TROPICAL DISEASES

Dr. Keith E. Evans

[1973]

If found, please ring 01.393.4656 or Kingston Hospital
(01.546.7711)

The Authors

FREDERICK J. WRIGHT

M.A., M.D.Cantab., F.R.C.P.Edin., F.R.C.P.Lond., D.T.M. & H.Eng.

*Senior Lecturer in Diseases of Tropical Climates, University of Edinburgh
Physician-in-charge Tropical Diseases Unit, City Hospital, Edinburgh
Consulting Physician to the Ministry of Overseas Development
Formerly Government Medical Specialist, Kenya*

JAMES P. BAIRD

M.D., F.R.C.P.Edin., F.R.C.P.Lond.

*Major-General, late R.A.M.C., Commandant and Director of Studies to
the Royal Army Medical College, Recently Consulting Physician to the British
Army, Professor of Military Medicine of the Royal Army Medical College and the
Royal College of Physicians, London
Formerly Officer-in-charge Medical Division, British Military Hospital, Singapore*

Supplement to

THE PRINCIPLES AND PRACTICE OF MEDICINE

Tenth Edition Edited by

SIR STANLEY DAVIDSON

and

JOHN MACLEOD

TROPICAL DISEASES

BY

FREDERICK J. WRIGHT

AND

JAMES P. BAIRD

FOURTH EDITION
REPRINT

CHURCHILL LIVINGSTONE
EDINBURGH & LONDON
1972

First Edition	1964
Reprinted	1965
First E.L.B.S. Edition	1965
Second Edition	1967
Second E.L.B.S. Edition	1967
Third Edition	1968
Third E.L.B.S. Edition	1968
Fourth Edition	1971
Reprinted	1972
Fourth E.L.B.S. Edition	1971
Reprinted	1972
Reprinted	1972

ISBN 0 443 00797 7

Printed in Great Britain

Preface to the Fourth Edition

THE *Tropical Diseases* Supplement to *The Principles and Practice of Medicine* has been very well received by students and doctors in the tropics. The reasons for excluding from it certain diseases which are described in the parent textbook are clearly stated in the preface to the first edition of the Supplement which is again recorded for the benefit of new readers.

Considerable progress has been made in tropical medicine since the printing of the third edition and every endeavour has been made to bring the text up to date by appropriate deletions and additions. Dr. N. C. Allan, Senior Lecturer in Haematology, University of Edinburgh (formerly of University of Ibadan, Nigeria) is now responsible for the section on Anaemia in the Tropics, succeeding Dr. Watson-Williams who has left the United Kingdom. The authors are much indebted to the following for expert advice on the subjects indicated: Drs. Stanley G. Browne (leprosy), A. D. M. Bryceson (cutaneous leishmaniasis and relapsing fever), Mr. Denis P. Burkitt (Burkitt's tumour), Dr. R. N. Chaudhuri (cholera), Professor L. H. Collier (trachoma), Mr. J. Cook (Kaposi's sarcoma), Dr. I. G. Murray (mycology), and Major R. N. T. Thin (melioidosis).

The authors also wish me to express their thanks to the many other colleagues who have given help and advice and to our publishers E. &. S. Livingstone for their kindly assistance and invaluable guidance throughout the preparation of the book.

STANLEY DAVIDSON

1971

Preface to the First Edition

THE *Principles and Practice of Medicine* has proved to be a popular textbook in many parts of the world. However, the valid criticism has been made by students and doctors in tropical countries that it did not include a description of many diseases of common occurrence and great importance to them. For students in temperate climates the inclusion of an account of these diseases would add unnecessarily to the size and scope of the book. Accordingly a supplement on tropical diseases has been written for those who practise in tropical countries. It is intended primarily for students and general practitioners living in the tropics and no attempt has been made by the authors to cover fully all aspects of tropical medicine. For further study, advanced books on tropical medicine or helminthology should be consulted.

I was fortunate in securing the services of the late Sir Alexander Biggam who, shortly before his lamented death, had completed the supplement in conjunction with Dr. Frederick J. Wright, Senior Lecturer, Diseases of Tropical Climates, in the University of Edinburgh. In addition, the section on Anaemia in the Tropics has been written by Dr. E. J. Watson-Williams, Lecturer in Clinical Haematology in the University of Manchester, an acknowledged authority in this field.

The following diseases, which are usually included in a textbook of tropical medicine, have been described in *The Principles and Practice of Medicine* because either they are sometimes encountered in practice in a temperate climate or they are of particular educational value. To avoid unnecessary repetition they have not been included in this Supplement.

* The page numbers refer to the tenth edition of *The Principles and Practice of Medicine*.

I am grateful to Dr. J. C. Gould and to the Oxford University Press for permission to reprint illustrations taken from *Medicine—the Diagnosis and*

Treatment of Prevalent Disease, by F. J. Wright and J. C. Gould, and to Brigadier L. S. R. Macfarlane for illustrations taken from *Human Proto-zoology and Helminthology*, published by E. &. S. Livingstone Ltd.

STANLEY DAVIDSON

1964

Contents

ix

Introduction

As stated in the preface to this Supplement, page vii, some important tropical diseases have already been described in *The Principles and Practice of Medicine* where some introductory comments and historical notes are also recorded (pp. **1112-1138**).

The conditions to be described below are grouped largely on an aetiological basis, beginning with further important protozoal infections. In the practice of tropical medicine it is, however, important to appreciate that an infecting agent may be only one factor in the malady produced. What transpires is often materially influenced by genetic endowment, inherited or acquired immunities, the nutritional state and the presence of concomitant diseases. Therefore it is better to think of the host-parasite relationship or the state of the patient in his environmental setting, rather than the characteristics of defined diseases. Similarly prevention and treatment are related primarily to the community or individual patient, not necessarily to the invading parasite. Nevertheless there are many specific infective agents responsible for ill-health in the tropics and, with the exception of the smaller viruses, the majority are amenable to specific chemotherapy if this can be taken to the patient. In any one locality it is prudent to learn what are the prevailing manifestations of endemic disorders. Thus the usual causes of splenomegaly, anaemia or jaundice may differ widely from place to place.

It may be noted that a few conditions, which occur only in temperate regions, have been included, e.g. rickettsialpox. This has been done to complete groups of diseases and to describe certain related conditions which have not been included in *The Principles and Practice of Medicine.*

1

Diseases due to Protozoa

LEISHMANIASES

THIS group of diseases is caused by protozoa of the genus *Leishmania*, conveyed to man by female sandflies in which the flagellate forms of leishmania are found. In man the leishmaniae are found in reticulo-endothelial cells in characteristic oval forms known as amastigotes or Leishman-Donovan (L.D.) bodies (Fig. 1). Leishmaniasis may take the form of a generalised infection called visceral leishmaniasis or kala azar. Localised lesions of the skin occur in cutaneous leishmaniasis or oriental sore. South American leishmaniasis may remain confined to the skin or progress to ulceration of mucous membranes. The causative leishmaniae are morphologically identical but differ in their serological reactions.

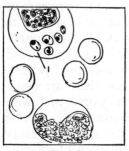

FIG. 1

1 Leishman-Donovan bodies.

Visceral Leishmaniasis
(Kala azar)

Kala azar is caused by *Leishmania donovani*.

Geographical Distribution. It is prevalent in the Mediterranean littoral, Ethiopia, Sudan, parts of East and West Africa, Asia Minor, mountainous regions of Southern Arabia, eastern parts of India, China and South America. In India man appears to be the chief host but in many areas, including the Mediterranean area, dogs are the main reservoir of infection. In the latter region the disease in local residents occurs chiefly in childhood, after which there is a degree of immunity.

Pathology. Multiplication, by simple fission, of leishmaniae takes place in reticulo-endothelial cells which rupture and the L.D. bodies are distributed to reticulo-endothelial cells in various organs, including the liver and spleen which become greatly enlarged. There is a marked progressive granulocytopenia, the leucocyte count often falling to 2,000/c.mm. or lower, and a slowly progressive anaemia. There is a great increase of gamma globulin. Successful chemotherapy reverses these changes; only rarely does appreciable fibrosis of the liver occur. Occasionally after recovery a condition of post-kala azar dermal leishmaniasis develops (see below).

Clinical Features. The incubation period of visceral leishmaniasis is usually about one or two months but exceptionally it may be prolonged

2

for years, up to 10 years having been recorded. The onset may be insidious or abrupt with sweating and high intermittent fever, sometimes showing a double rise of temperature in the 24 hours. The spleen and usually also the liver to a rather less degree soon become enlarged, the spleen, after some weeks, often reaching a great size. If not treated the patient will become anaemic and wasted, frequently with increased pigmentation especially on the face. Except in acute cases the patient may remain ambulant although febrile. Lymph nodes may be enlarged. Rarely lymphadenopathy is the only clinical abnormality. In India about 5 per cent. of cases, one to two years after apparent cure, develop post-kala azar dermal leishmaniasis. In some other countries this condition occurs less frequently but rather sooner. It may present first as hypopigmented or erythematous macules on any part of the body and later a nodular eruption may appear, especially on the face. In the macular lesions scanty intracellular L.D. bodies may be found. In nodules they are more abundant.

Diagnosis. The somewhat variable clinical picture of visceral leishmaniasis and leucopenia are usually supported by a high level of gamma globulin demonstrable by paper electrophoresis of the blood and responsible for the positive formol-gel test. The latter is carried out by adding 1 drop of commercial formalin to 1 ml. of the patient's serum. In an established case the serum becomes solid and opaque within 20 minutes. A complement-fixation test is available and an immunofluorescent test has been developed. The leishmaniae (as L.D. bodies) may be demonstrated by staining material obtained by puncture of sternal marrow or lymph node or, failing these, by puncture of the spleen or liver. Culture of blood or marrow aspirate on a special medium at room temperature may yield the flagellate forms of the leishmania after incubation for periods of one to three weeks. Kala azar has to be differentiated from typhoid fever and brucellosis, for the diagnosis of which agglutination tests and culture of the blood are employed, and from malaria by examination of blood films. The hepatosplenomegaly may be simulated by schistosomiasis. Tuberculosis, leukaemia and reticulosis may be incorrectly suspected. Any of these conditions, but especially those due to endemic infections, may be present in addition to kala azar. Post-kala azar dermal leishmaniasis has to be distinguished from leprosy, yaws, syphilis, lupus vulgaris, drug sensitivity and other dermatoses.

Treatment. The response to treatment varies with the geographical area in which the disease has been acquired. In India the disease is readily cured, but in the Sudan and East Africa it is more resistant. Sodium stibogluconate, a pentavalent antimony compound, gives good results. A solution containing 100 mg./ml. is available for intravenous or intramuscular use. A suitable course of treatment for an adult is 10 daily intravenous injections of 600 mg. repeated, if necessary, after an interval of 14 days up to a total dosage of 12 or even 18 g. Children tolerate a relatively larger dose of antimony than adults and seem to require it. One-third of the adult dose may be given to children from 5 to 10 years of age.

The diamidine compounds, pentamidine isethionate employed as in trypanosomiasis (p. 10) and 2-hydroxystilbamidine isethionate, have been found useful in some areas where the disease is resistant to treatment with antimony compounds. The dose of 2-hydroxystilbamidine for an adult is 250 mg. intravenously daily for 10 days; the course may be repeated after an interval of 14 days up to a total of 7·5 g. given over a period of 58 days. Side-effects such as fever, rigors and headache are not uncommon with this treatment but can be relieved by giving 10 mg. of mepyramine maleate three times a day during the course.

The results produced in each case must be assessed and treatment continued as required. Favourable signs are absence of fever, increase in weight, improvement of the anaemia, a normal white cell count, return towards normal level of serum gamma globulin, recession of the spleen and negative lymph node puncture. For the treatment of post-kala azar dermal leishmaniasis the same drugs are used as for visceral leishmaniasis but the response is slower, and intermittent treatment for months may be required. Some respond well to pentamidine isethionate. A generous diet should be given and any concomitant disease treated.

Prophylaxis. In an endemic area infected dogs should be destroyed. Sandflies should be combated (p. 52). Treatment of human infections reduces their infectivity for sandflies.

Cutaneous Leishmaniasis (Oriental Sore)

Oriental sore, which is caused by *Leishmania tropica* is widespread in the tropics and subtropics. It is conveyed from many different animals to man by certain species of sandflies after the leishmaniae have undergone a cycle of development in these insects.

Pathology. In the early stages, before ulceration, there is a granulomatous reaction in the corium consisting of lymphocytes, plasma cells and numerous hypertrophic reticulo-endothelial cells, some of which are packed with leishmaniae. As the process extends, the epithelium becomes thinned and the raised papule ulcerates in the centre and later suffers pyogenic infection. The margin of the ulcer consists of dense epithelial proliferation and in the centre the whole thickness of the skin is destroyed. The base of the ulcer consists of granulomatous cells. Considerable scarring may result, especially where there has been marked secondary infection.

Clinical Features. The incubation period is from two weeks to five or more years but usually is from two to three months. Lesions, single or multiple on exposed parts of the body, start as small itchy red papules and with increase in size a scab forms on the surface. Untreated this will progress to form a rounded ulcer with well-defined indurated raised margins and a granulomatous base. These lesions may be up to 10 cm. or more in diameter. A seropurulent discharge exudes which may dry and form an adherent scab. Pain is not a feature and general symptoms are usually absent. Sometimes, instead of an ulcer, a fungating nodular mass develops. Occasionally leishmaniae spread from the sore and these cause nodules to develop in the course of the lymphatics with enlargement of the related nodes. Untreated the ulcer lasts about a year. Immunity has by then developed and this will prevent further infection. After healing a thin depressed depigmented scar remains. Cutaneous leishmaniasis may occur in a persistent relapsing form (leishmaniasis recidiva) having a tuberculoid histology.

Diffuse cutaneous leishmaniasis occurring in Ethiopia and Venezuela is probably attributable to a defective host reaction to *L. tropica*. After the initial lesion diffuse hypertrophic lesions develop and, untreated, spread inexorably to involve much of the body. The lesions contain numerous L.D. bodies engulfed by macrophages.

Diagnosis. The appearance of the lesion in a patient from an endemic area suggests the diagnosis. Leishman-Donovan bodies can be demonstrated by inserting a dry needle into the margin of the ulcer or curetting the edge and staining the material obtained with Giemsa's stain or culturing it on a special medium at room temperature. A Leishmanin (Montenegro) skin test (p. 7) is positive except in untreated diffuse cutaneous leishmaniasis. Other localised skin lesions such as those of rodent ulcer, yaws, leprosy and primary syphilis have to be differentiated.

Treatment. An important part of the general treatment in long-standing cases is the cleansing of the ulcer. The crust should be removed by the application of moist dressings and the exposed surface then kept clean. In addition it may be necessary to administer an antibiotic if secondary pyogenic infection is present.

Specific treatment to eradicate the leishmaniae is given either locally or parenterally, the choice being influenced by the number and distribution of the lesions. For only one or at the most three lesions, local treatment is often successful. Unipolar coagulation diathermy has replaced earlier methods of inducing an inflammatory reaction.

When the lesions are multiple it is better to treat the patient by parenteral injections of pentavalent antimony compounds such as sodium stibogluconate as prescribed for visceral leishmaniasis (p. 3), and this, combined with local cleansing of the lesion, is also preferable for a solitary lesion on the face. Some lesions are relatively resistant and require prolonged antimony therapy. A useful alternative is oral dehydroemetine. This is presented as the dihydrochloride or resinate. The dose is 3 to 4·5 mg./kg. body weight, daily, in three divided doses, for four weeks.

Diffuse cutaneous leishmaniasis responds poorly to antimonials. Cure can usually be achieved by repeated courses of intramuscular pentamidine isethionate (p. 10) but weekly glucose tolerance tests are required to detect the early signs of drug-induced diabetes. Response may also be obtained to intravenous amphotericin B (p. 102). With successful treatment the Leishmanin skin test becomes positive and the lesions fibrose.

Prophylaxis. In addition to those preventive measures described under visceral leishmaniasis against animals and sandflies, a lasting immunity can be achieved by deliberate inoculation of a living culture of *L. tropica*. This produces an ulcer, but the site chosen for the inoculation is one normally covered by clothing so scarring does not cause undesirable disfigurement. This procedure does not protect against visceral leishmaniasis for which no effective vaccine has been prepared.

South American Leishmaniasis

South American leishmaniasis has in the past been attributed to *Leishmania braziliensis* but several different species or sub-species are now recognised, namely *L. braziliensis*, *L. mexicana* and *L. peruviana*. They occur only in hot, moist, afforested regions and are conveyed to man from a variety of animals by several species of sandflies. The disease can be separated into three types. There is the 'espundia' of Brazil caused by *L. braziliensis*. Secondly there is the 'chicleros ulcer' or 'bay sore' attributable to *L. mexicana* found in Mexico, Guatemala and Honduras among gatherers of chicle, used for making chewing gum. The third variety is the disease occurring in the Guianas and Peru, known as 'uta' and caused by *L. peruviana*. Diffuse cutaneous leishmaniasis was attributed in Venezuela to a distinct species *L. americana* or *L. pifanoi*. It may be an abnormal host reaction to *L. tropica* (p. 5).

Geographical Distribution. The infections are endemic in Central and South American countries and in parts of Mexico.

Pathology. The microscopic appearances of the skin lesions may be similar to oriental sore but are not always characteristic and diagnosis may therefore have to depend on the demonstration of the parasite, which is often difficult. The mucocutaneous lesions begin as a perivascular infiltration; later endarteritis may lead to destruction of the surrounding tissues (see below).

Clinical Features. In the classical espundia of Brazil and surrounding regions the initial papulo-pustular cutaneous lesions may be localised or widespread and affect especially the face, ears, elbows and knees. Mucosal lesions either accompany the skin lesions or appear some years later. The nasal mucosa becomes congested and later all tissues of the nose ulcerate except for the bone. The lips, soft palate and fauces may be invaded and destroyed leading to terrible suffering and deformity. Secondary bacterial infection is a common aggravating factor.

Chicleros ulcers affect mostly the ears and the lesions often last many years. They start as small painless pimples which enlarge to become larger papules going on to ulceration and erosion of the pinna. The lesions of uta rarely progress beyond the skin. They are often multiple and papillomatous rather than ulcerative.

Diagnosis. This depends on the history and clinical appearance, confirmed by demonstration of the protozoon by punch biopsy. As parasites are not easily found the Leishmanin (Montenegro) test is of value. In this an antigen prepared from a culture of leishmaniae is used and 0·1 ml. of this is injected intradermally. A positive case will show erythema and induration at the site of the injection after 48 hours. South American leishmaniasis has to be distinguished from leprosy, yaws and various fungal diseases.

Treatment. Early cases and those exhibiting chicleros ulcers may be successfully treated by sodium stibogluconate given as recommended for visceral leishmaniasis (p. 3). In more advanced cases amphotericin B, although a toxic drug, given by intravenous infusion as for histoplasmosis (p. 102) may succeed. Pyrimethamine, given orally, has also been used successfully. Three courses, each lasting 10 days, are given, separated by rest periods of 8 days. In the first two courses the daily dose is 50 mg.; in the third it is reduced to 25 mg.

AFRICAN TRYPANOSOMIASIS
(Sleeping Sickness)

African sleeping sickness is caused by trypanosomes conveyed to man by the bites of infected tsetse flies of either sex.

Geographical Distribution. The disease is acquired only in Africa between 12° N. and 25° S. There are two trypanosomes which affect man, *Trypanosoma gambiense* conveyed by *Glossina palpalis* and *G. tachinoides* and *T. rhodesiense* transmitted by *G. morsitans*, *G. pallidipes*, *G. swynnertoni* and also *G. palpalis*. Gambiense trypanosomiasis has a wide distribution in West and Central Africa reaching to Uganda and Kenya; rhodesiense trypanosomiasis is found in parts of East and Central Africa. *G. palpalis* is found only on or near the shady banks of lakes and streams; *G. tachinoides* travels farther afield. *G. swynnertoni* is limited to Tanzania and, in common with other vectors of rhodesiense sleeping sickness, flies across open country covered with scrub. In these areas wild animals are found commonly to be affected by other trypanosomes, such as *T. vivax*, *T. congolense* and *T. brucei* which also cause much sickness among cattle. These trypanosomes thus indirectly affect man by reducing greatly the grazing areas on which cattle can survive, thus reducing supplies of milk and meat, prime requirements for the prevention of protein malnutrition. *T. brucei* has not been distinguished morphologically or antigenically from *T. rhodesiense* but only the latter is pathogenic for man. On epidemiological grounds it appears that there is undoubtedly a reservoir of infection of *T. rhodesiense* in wild animals and, at times, in cattle. Experimental transmission of *T. rhodesiense* to man from a bushbuck has been achieved but this does not establish that this animal is the most important reservoir host. There is also evidence that at times *T. gambiense* may be harboured by cattle. It is arguable whether *T. gambiense* and *T. rhodesiense* should be regarded as different species or as divergent strains of one species.

Pathological and Clinical Features. Even during an epidemic of trypanosomiasis, only a low percentage of tsetse flies are infected. A bite by a tsetse fly is frequently painful but, if trypanosomes are introduced, the site of the bite may again become painful and swollen about 10 days later. The lesion is sometimes described as a 'trypanosomal chancre'. Trypanosomes can be recovered from it. Within two to three weeks of infection the trypanosomes invade the blood stream. In gambiense infections the disease usually runs a relatively slow course with irregular bouts of moderate fever and enlargement of lymphatic nodes. These are characteristically firm, discrete, rubbery and painless and are particularly prominent in the posterior triangle of the neck. Sometimes during these early weeks transient circinate erythematous eruptions can be seen, particularly on the front or back of the chest and especially if the patient has a white skin. Bouts of fever lasting a week or more recur over a period of months and tachycardia persists in the apyrexial intervals. The spleen and liver may become palpable. Varying degrees of chronicity may be encountered and signs and symptoms may be few. After some months, in the absence of treatment, the central nervous system is invaded. This is shown clinically by headaches and changed behaviour, insomnia by night and sleepiness by day, mental confusion and eventually tremors, pareses, wasting from inanition, coma and death. The earliest sign of invasion of the nervous system is an increase of protein and cells in the cerebrospinal fluid. The histological changes in the brain are similar to those found in viral encephalitis but trypanosomes are scattered in the substance of the brain and large eosinophilic mononuclear cells with a deeply stained oval eccentric nucleus (morula cells) are a feature. Sometimes gambiense infections run a more acute course resembling the illness more typical of rhodesiense trypanosomiasis.

In rhodesiense infections enlargement of the lymph nodes is not a prominent feature. Fever is higher and more constant than in gambiense infections, so that within a few weeks the patient is severely ill and may have developed pleural effusions and signs of myocarditis. The clinical manifestations of involvement of the nervous system may not be obvious but within a few weeks of infection the cerebrospinal fluid will be abnormal and in the untreated case death ensues from toxaemia or heart failure, often with complicating factors such as pneumonia or dysentery. If the illness is a little less acute, tremors, drowsiness and coma may develop.

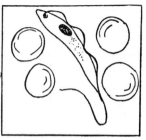

Fig. 2

Trypanosome in blood film.

Diagnosis. In any febrile patient from an endemic area trypanosomiasis should be considered. In rhodesiense infections the trypanosomes can usually be detected by microscopic examination of a wet blood film. Agitation of red cells by the trypanosomes is seen and staining of thick and thin blood films, as for the detection of malaria, will reveal trypanosomes. Where necessary concentration methods, with centrifuged citrated specimens of blood, should be used. In the earliest stages of gambiense infections the trypanosomes may be seen in the blood or from puncture of the primary lesion but it is usually easier to demonstrate them by puncture of a lymph node. Using a medium sized dry needle, the node, held between finger and thumb, is punctured and the node moved on the needle and the material aspirated and examined in a similar way to the blood. Animal inoculation and culture on a special medium can also be employed. A complement-fixation test with an antigen from *T. equiperdum* has been used to detect relapses of *T. gambiense* infections. Trypanosomes are only occasionally found in the cerebrospinal fluid but examination of it is an important routine measure to assess, by the cell count and especially the protein content, the degree of affection, if any, of the nervous system.

Except in cases with undoubted established neurological abnormalities, lumbar puncture should be deferred until the first dose of a trypanocidal drug has been given. This will reduce the risk of implantation of trypanosomes into the cerebrospinal fluid, by the lumbar puncture needle.

Treatment. If treatment is begun early, before the brain has been invaded, it will be curative. For this purpose either suramin or pentamidine isethionate may be used, the latter being employed only for gambiense infections. After the nervous system is affected an arsenical will be required as suramin and pentamidine do not penetrate into the brain. Tryparsamide was formerly used widely but the arsenicals now recommended are melarsoprol or melarsonyl potassium.

Suramin, a complex organic urea compound, is usually given intravenously. An initial trial dose of 200 mg. is given to test for sensitivity. This is followed on the next day by 1 g. dissolved in 10 ml. of distilled water repeated at intervals of three to five days to a total dosage of 5 to 10 g. Children tolerate the drug well, the adult dose of 1 g. being reduced for a child under 3 years to 250 mg. and from 3 to 10 years to 500 mg. given in a course similar to that recommended for adults. Toxic effects which may occur include dermatitis, nausea, vomiting and peripheral neuritis. Also, as the kidneys may be affected the urine should be examined before each injection and the drug discontinued if red cells and casts appear.

Pentamidine isethionate, an aromatic diamidine, is less toxic than suramin. It is rather painful when administered intramuscularly but, as there may be sudden collapse from a rapid fall in blood pressure when the drug is used intravenously, this route is not recommended. The intramuscular dose is 3 to 5 mg./kg. body weight to a maximum of 250 mg. dissolved in 5 ml. distilled water, on alternate days for 10 injections.

Melarsoprol is a chemical combination of the trivalent melarsan oxide and dimercaprol. It is presented as a 3·6 per cent. w/v solution in glycol-propylene and is administered intravenously. Although a toxic drug, it has proved highly efficacious in advanced rhodesiense infections, which were formerly fatal, and for other resistant and relapsing cases. The main danger is encephalopathy due to a Jarisch-Herxheimer reaction to the death of many trypanosomes. Before commencing treatment with melarsoprol the patient's general condition may be benefited by a few preliminary injections of suramin. The initial dose of melarsoprol is assessed on the patient's general condition rather than on his weight. Patients who are severely ill may at first only tolerate as small a dose as 0·5 ml. of the 3·6 per cent. w/v solution and the initial dose must never exceed 2 ml. Further injections are given on the second and third days. The maximum dose is 3·6 mg./kg. body weight, i.e. 5 ml. of 3·6 per cent. w/v solution for a man of 50 kg. There then follows a rest period of one to two weeks followed by a second series of three injections. If the initial dose was very small, additional courses may be required during the next four or five weeks. The total dosage aimed at is 30 ml. of the 3·6 per cent. w/v solution. Melarsoprol should only be given under medical supervision.

Melarsonyl potassium (Trimelarsan) is a water-soluble derivative of melarsoprol suitable for intramuscular injection. It is less toxic than melarsoprol. The daily dose is 4 mg./kg. body weight administered as follows. As a test for sensitivity a half dose is given, followed by three successive full daily doses. For intermediate and late cases, after an interval of 7 to 10 days a further four daily doses are given. Good results have been obtained in gambiense trypanosomiasis. It is not a fully reliable drug for rhodesiense infections.

Nitrofurazone is liable to produce undesirable side-effects including haemolytic anaemia in those whose red cells are deficient in glucose-6-phosphate dehydrogenase but has occasionally been successful. It should only be used when all other drugs have failed. The adult dose is 500 mg. orally three times daily for 10 days.

GENERAL MEASURES. Malnutrition and any concomitant infection should be combated.

Personal Prophylaxis. Against *T. gambiense* a single intramuscular injection of 250 mg. pentamidine gives protection for six months because of the slow excretion of the drug. As the protection against *T. rhodesiense* is less sure and shorter in duration, chemoprophylaxis is not advised in rhodesiense areas as the infection may be masked until a late stage is reached. In such areas it is safer to have no protection but to ensure early recognition of the 'trypanosomal chancre' and to have the blood examined at monthly intervals or whenever there is any fever. Prompt treatment will then be curative.

AMERICAN TRYPANOSOMIASIS
(Chagas' Disease)

The cause of Chagas' disease is *Trypanosoma cruzi* transmitted to man from the faeces of a reduviid bug in which the trypanosomes have a cycle of development before becoming infective to man. They enter through the conjunctiva, mucosa of mouth or nose or through an abrasion of the skin. The bugs are liable to fly down from the ceilings of primitive houses on to the faces of those sleeping below. Dogs and cats are the most important hosts in nature although many wild and domestic animals may harbour the infection. Acute illness has also followed transfusion of infected blood.

Pathology. At the site of entry there is usually a local tissue reaction. The trypanosomes travel by the blood stream and develop into leishmanoid forms. These are liable to multiply in the myocardium causing pseudocysts in the muscle fibres and also in the nervous system, giving rise to the changes described below.

Clinical Features. The entrance of *T. cruzi* through an abrasion produces a dusky-red firm swelling with enlargement of regional lymph nodes. Although less common, a conjunctival lesion is more pathognomonic; the unilateral firm reddish swelling of the lids may close the eye and constitutes 'Romana's sign'. Evidence of a generalised infection soon appears, young children being the most severely affected with the temperature rising to 40° C. (104° F.) and lasting for two weeks or more. Tachycardia, always a feature, may persist for months. In addition to generalised lymphadenopathy there may also be enlargement of the spleen and liver. Neurological features include insomnia, personality changes and signs of meningo-encephalitis. Chronic infections frequently damage Auerbach's plexus with resulting dilatation of various parts of the alimentary canal, especially the colon and even including the appendix. Dilatation of the bile ducts and bronchi are also recognised sequelae. Invasion of the myocardium causes a cardiomyopathy (p. 336) as indicated by cardiac dilatation, dysrhythmias and partial or complete heart block. Only infants die readily from the acute infection, death being caused in the first few days of the illness by encephalitis or a few weeks later by myocarditis or an overwhelming generalised infection. In those who survive the acute phase the trypanosomes often persist, causing a chronic illness from which a slow recovery takes place. Many cases are difficult to diagnose because there may be no apparent site of entry and there may be no acute phase. Chagas' disease is being increasingly recognised, in the endemic areas, as a cause of cardiomyopathy, responsible, on occasion, for sudden death particularly in adult males during exercise.

Diagnosis. A history of residence in an endemic area with suggestive symptoms indicates the need for a search for *T. cruzi* in the blood or for the leishmanoid forms in other tissues. The trypanosomes are often scanty in the blood but may be recovered by culture. Xenodiagnosis has been used with success. In this method infection-free, laboratory-bred, reduviid bugs are fed on the patient and two weeks later and subsequently for periods up to one year the hind gut or faeces of the bug are examined for metacyclic trypanosomes. A complement-fixation test (Guerreiro-Machado reaction) has also been used as a means of diagnosis. In acute cases a positive result can be expected but in chronic infections the results are disappointing.

Treatment. No fully effective specific remedy is available. Arsenobenzyl sulphate is used in the hope of slowing down the progress of the infection. It is given in a 10 per cent. solution beginning with 150 mg. for an adult, increasing gradually to 450 mg. up to a total of 5 g. An alternative which is used is tetracycline, 2 g. daily in divided doses, combined with primaquine 7·5 mg. base twice daily, both for 14 days.

Prevention. Preventive measures should include improved housing and destruction of reduviid bugs by spraying of houses with lindane (gamma BHC).

BALANTIDIASIS

Balantidium coli, a large ciliate protozoon, affects pigs and occasionally man.

Geographical Distribution. The infection is seen, but only infrequently, in all countries among those who tend domestic pigs.

Pathology. The pathology is similar to that of intestinal amoebiasis. *Balantidium coli* may live free in the lumen of the bowel or it may cause ulceration in the colon; in severe cases almost the whole extent of the lower bowel may be affected and also the lower part of the ileum.

Clinical Features. The infection may be symptomless but when ulceration occurs frequent stools are passed together with blood and mucus.

Diagnosis. *Balantidium coli* is recognised in the stool by microscopic examination.

Treatment. The disease usually responds to the arsenical Carbarsone, 250 mg. given orally twice daily for 10 days. Other cases respond better to tetracycline 0·5 g. four times daily for 10 days. In debilitated persons the disease may become chronic and the infection may be difficult to eradicate.

GIARDIASIS
(Flagellate Diarrhoea)

The human infection is due to *Giardia intestinalis*, a pear-shaped flagellate 12 to 18 microns in length.

Geographical Distribution. It is world-wide in its distribution but more common in the tropics.

Pathology. The flagellates inhabit the small intestine and cause a mild enteritis.

Clinical Features. The infection is often symptomless but recurrent attacks of urgent diarrhoea with abdominal discomfort and loose pale stools are characteristic. In heavy infections there may be evidence of malabsorption.

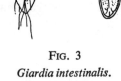

Diagnosis. The symptoms might suggest sprue or intestinal amoebiasis but the flagellates, or during quiescent periods their cysts, are found on microscopic examination of the stool.

FIG. 3

Giardia intestinalis.
Vegetative and cystic forms.

Treatment. Mepacrine 100 mg. or alternatively metronidazole 200 mg. three times daily after food for seven days is given to an adult and the course may need to be repeated after a free interval of one week. Children under four years of age can be given one-quarter of the adult dose and from four to eight years half of the adult dose, of either drug.

TOXOPLASMOSIS

Toxoplasmosis is caused by *Toxoplasma gondii*, a small protozoon. Human infection after birth may be acquired from a wide variety of birds and mammals. Transmission from mother to foetus causes congenital toxoplasmosis.

Geographical Distribution. Human toxoplasmosis occurs widely in North, Central and South America, Europe, Asia and Africa.

Pathology. In the congenital form the organism is widespread in the central nervous system, eyes, heart, lungs and adrenals. If the infant survives, the parasite soon disappears from most organs except the central nervous system and eyes. The brain shows large areas of necrosis with cyst formation and patchy calcification; the spinal cord may be similarly affected. In adults the lesions, confined largely to the lung, may produce areas of fibrosis.

Clinical Features. The manifestations in congenital infections are mainly cerebral. There may be hydrocephalus or microcephaly associated with convulsions, tremors or paralysis with resultant contractures. Radiological examination may show patches of calcification in the brain. Eye defects, microphthalmos, nystagmus and chorio-retinitis are common. The cerebrospinal fluid is often xanthochromic with increased protein and mononuclear cells. An enlarged liver, jaundice, diminished thrombo-cytes and purpura may also be found. Congenital infections are usually fatal, and if the child survives he is usually gravely incapacitated.

In acquired infections symptoms are more variable. Many are symptom-less. In the acute form there may be pneumonitis with fever, cough, generalised aches and pains and inconstantly a maculopapular rash. In the more chronic infections, often afebrile, there may be only enlargement of the lymph nodes with a lymphocytosis showing atypical mononuclear cells similar to those present in infectious mononucleosis. Toxoplasmosis is recognised as a cause of chorio-retinitis and uveitis in adults.

Diagnosis. In congenital toxoplasmosis the neurological signs and symptoms suggest the diagnosis. The mothers from whom the infection is transmitted have symptomless infections. Serological tests are of value in indicating the presence of active or past infections. The dye test (Sabin and Feldman) becomes positive early in the disease and persists for years. This test depends on the finding that toxoplasma incubated with normal serum stain with methylene blue, whereas if they are incubated with serum containing antibodies they do not stain. The occurrence of positive tests in those free from symptoms necessitates caution in their interpreta-tion in relation to an individual clinical problem. Biopsy material, such as that obtained from a lymph node, may yield the *Toxoplasma* on culture or by inoculation of a laboratory animal.

Treatment. A combination of a sulphonamide 1 g. six-hourly and pyrimethamine 25 mg. daily for two weeks has been shown to be beneficial in the treatment of chorio-retinitis due to toxoplasmosis and should be administered in all active cases.

Diseases due to Bacteria, Spirochaetes and Spirilla

GRANULOMA VENEREUM
(Ulcerating Granuloma of the Pudenda, Donovanosis)

GRANULOMA venereum is a venereal disease due to *Klebsiella granulomatis*, characterised by intracellular Donovan bodies, 1 to 2 microns in size, demonstrable in the endothelial and mononuclear cells of the lesion.

The disease has a wide distribution throughout the tropics and subtropics.

Pathology. At the margin of the lesion there is infiltration of the superficial portion of the corium and of the papillae by lymphocytes and mononuclear cells in which Donovan bodies can be demonstrated. Excessive fibrous tissue is formed especially in lesions of long standing.

Clinical Features. The incubation period is variable, from a few days to three months after exposure. The primary lesion is a small nodule or papule in the skin or mucous membrane of the external genitalia. This progresses to form a superficial serpiginous ulcer spreading peripherally. Auto-infection of an opposing surface also extends the spread. Moist warm areas of the body, particularly the flexures of the thighs, the folds between the scrotum and thighs in the male and the labia and vagina in the female, are especially vulnerable. The perianal region and occasionally the face and mucous membrane of the mouth, in addition to the genital area, may also be affected. Untreated, the lesions may continue for years, spreading at the periphery and leaving an unhealthy central scarred area which tends to break down from slight trauma.

Healing of the ulcer is often associated with excessive fibrous tissue formation which may lead to scarring and stenosis of the urethra, anal orifice or vagina. The lymph nodes, however, are not affected, and constitutional symptoms are slight or absent. A few cases of generalised donovanosis have been reported.

Diagnosis. A chronic superficial spreading ulcer in the genital region without any enlargement of the lymph nodes should suggest the disease; the detection of Donovan bodies is diagnostic.

Treatment. Streptomycin 1 g. daily for 7 to 14 days intramuscularly or tetracycline for 10 days orally is the treatment of choice. Surgery may be needed to alleviate the effects of scarring.

BARTONELLOSIS
(Carrión's Disease, Oroya Fever, Verruga Peruana)

This disease is caused by a small organism, *Bartonella bacilliformis*, transmitted by sandflies.

Geographical Distribution. It is prevalent in narrow hot valleys on the western slopes of the Andes at heights between 2,000 and 10,000 feet. Thus it is found in Peru, Ecuador, Bolivia, Colombia and Chile. The distribution coincides with the presence of the sandflies, *Phlebotomus verrucarum* and *P. noguchi*, but it is possible that the disease may also be transmitted by lice and ticks.

Pathology. In the acute form of the disease, Oroya fever, there is severe haemolysis. The spleen, liver and lymph nodes are enlarged. The bone marrow shows normoblastic hyperplasia, but megaloblastic changes have also been described presumably due to folic acid deficiency. Bartonellae are present in large numbers, often in clumps, in the erythrocytes and also in the endothelial cells lining the small vessels of the spleen, lymph nodes, adrenals, kidneys, bone marrow and elsewhere. There are necrotic foci in the liver and spleen. In the later stage of the disease, verruga peruana, cutaneous nodules form, microscopically resembling haemangiomas but containing scanty bartonellae in the endothelial cells.

Clinical Features. After an incubation period of 14 to 21 days the early stage, Oroya fever, develops with a sudden rise of temperature to 40° C. (104° F.) and rapid haemolysis leading to progressive pallor and prostration. The fever is accompanied by pains in muscles and joints, nausea, vomiting and diarrhoea and may terminate in delirium and coma. The red cell count may fall to one million in four days. Bartonellae are seen in stained blood films and in severe infections over 90 per cent. of the erythrocytes contain from 1 to 50 or more organisms. The anaemia is macro-normoblastic, with anisocytosis, poikilocytosis and polychromatophilia and many reticulocytes, normoblasts and a pronounced neutrophil leucocytosis. The spleen and liver are enlarged and tender. Secondary infection by salmonellae is a frequent cause of death. The first stage lasts from one to three weeks. In those who survive, the bartonellae soon disappear and the destroyed red cells are rapidly replaced. Cultures of the blood taken over a period of months may, however, continue to yield the organisms. Untreated the mortality in the acute form of the disease, especially prevalent in children, is over 90 per cent.

The cutaneous form, verruga peruana, usually follows 30 to 40 days after the febrile phase but occasionally there is no preceding fever. The eruption consists of cherry-red haemangioma-like cutaneous nodules 2 to 10 mm. in diameter. They are distributed peripherally on the head and limbs. Occasionally there may be a number on the mucous membrane of the mouth and pharynx. The cutaneous lesions are oval or rounded and lie half-buried in the skin. They are covered with a bluish epidermis which may ulcerate after slight injury. These lesions often appear in crops but they heal completely in two to three months. This stage is never fatal.

Diagnosis. The diagnosis is suggested by the clinical picture in an endemic area and is confirmed by the demonstration of bartonellae in the erythrocytes. In the verruga stage the organisms are found in the endothelial cells in biopsy tissue. Blood cultures may be positive in both stages.

Treatment. In the early febrile stage penicillin, streptomycin or tetracycline for five days give good results. Blood transfusions, fluids and electrolytes may be urgently required. If the anaemia is megaloblastic hydroxocobalamin or folic acid should be given (p. **846**). The cutaneous lesions require no local treatment except, occasionally, haemostasis.

Personal Protection. The use of insecticides, insect repellents and suitable protective clothing is advisable (p. 52).

MELIOIDOSIS

Melioidosis is caused by *Pseudomonas pseudomallei*, a micro-organism closely related to *Ps. mallei*, the cause of glanders, which is a rare disease of horses and grooms. *Ps. pseudomallei* is found in puddles following recent rain which suggests it may be saprophytic in nature. Observations suggest that many infections are acquired through abrasions of the skin although the respiratory and alimentary routes may also be possible. Diabetics and patients with severe burns are particularly vulnerable to infection.

Geographical Distribution. The disease has been increasingly reported from the Far East and Malaysia but also from Africa, Australia and elsewhere.

Pathology. A bacteraemia results in the formation of abscesses in the lungs, liver and spleen. In more chronic forms multiple abscesses continue to recur in subcutaneous tissue in addition to internal organs.

Clinical Features. In the majority there are high fever, prostration and signs of pneumonitis, with enlargement of the liver and spleen and sometimes dysenteric symptoms. A radiograph of the lungs resembles that of acute caseous tuberculosis. In the chronic forms multiple abscesses develop.

Diagnosis. The disease may be suspected from the clinical and radiographic appearances, and in acute cases blood culture or culture of the sputum may yield *Ps. pseudomallei* which can also be recovered from abscesses in the more chronic disease. Except in fulminating infections antibodies, which are common also to those produced in glanders, may be detected by agglutination and complement-fixation tests. A haemagglutination test is more sensitive and is specific for *Ps. pseudomallei*.

Treatment. Prompt treatment, without waiting for cultural confirmation, with tetracycline 3 g. daily or carbenicillin in large doses daily, has cured some early cases and these antibiotics or a sulphonamide as indicated by sensitivity tests assist recovery from more chronic infections. In addition, if subcutaneous or deep abscesses have developed their drainage is required.

LEPROSY

Leprosy is a chronic granulomatous disease caused by *Mycobacterium leprae*, an acid- and alcohol-fast organism that resembles *Myco. tuberculosis* in many ways. Widespread lesions of lepromatous leprosy have been reproduced in irradiated and thymectomised mice. Local multiplication of the organism in the foot-pads of mice is proving a most useful technique for demonstrating the identity and viability of *Myco. leprae* and the existence of drug-resistant strains, the screening of drugs, the effect of B.C.G. vaccination, and for the study of cell-mediated immunity. The mode of entry of *Myco. leprae* into the body has not been conclusively proved; it is generally assumed that the organism may pass through damaged skin or respiratory mucosa. Most patients give a history of prolonged association, especially in childhood or adolescence, with someone suffering from an open form of leprosy. The silent (or incubation) period is usually between two and five years.

Geographical Distribution. The disease is common in tropical Asia, the Far East, tropical Africa, Central and South America, and in some Pacific Islands, and the total number of people affected with leprosy is estimated at 15 million.

Pathology. The organisms show a predilection for nerve tissue, skin and the mucosa of the upper respiratory tract. The reaction of the host to their presence varies within the widest limits. In *tuberculoid leprosy* there is a marked cellular response, indicative of a vigorous defence, around nerves, sweat glands and hair follicles. Organisms are scanty, and found mainly in the vicinity of terminal nerve endings in the dermis. They are seen only after prolonged search or by the use of concentration techniques. Lymphocytes, histiocytes and epithelial cells, some coalescing to form giant cells, are grouped in foci resembling tubercles. In contrast to the typical picture in lepromatous leprosy, the cellular infiltration may extend to and through the subepidermal zone. Tuberculoid leprosy is usually considered to be non-infective.

In *lepromatous leprosy*, the infective form of the disease, organisms are present in great abundance in the dermis, eventually replacing the normal architecture. They are mainly grouped in 'globi', which are large macrophages containing 50 or more organisms, and are found in nerve tissue, the arrectores pilorum muscles and the endothelial cells of blood vessels; rarely in the cells of the epidermis itself. They are carried in the blood stream (in which they can be demonstrated) to distant and deep organs including lymph nodes, bone marrow, Kupffer cells of the liver and the spleen. Terminal amyloid disease is not uncommon.

Between these two 'polar' types of leprosy, there are diverse intermediate manifestations grouped under the terms '*borderline*' or '*dimorphous*'. The host reaction varies within wide limits from the near-lepromatous to the near-tuberculoid; it may vary also from time to time in the same patient. The early infection, usually transient, and either self-healing or giving place to one or other of the determinate types, is called '*indeterminate*'. The histological appearances in it are non-specific, and consist of groups of round cells diffusely scattered in the dermis. *Myco. leprae* are demonstrable in varying numbers in borderline and indeterminate leprosy. The differing tissue response is usually paralleled by the reaction in the lepromin test which determines sensitivity to an intradermal injection of a sterilised extract of lepromatous tissue. Positive reactions are obtained in tuberculoid leprosy, a negative response in lepromatous leprosy and negative or weak positive responses in indeterminate and borderline leprosy. This test is of no value in establishing the diagnosis of leprosy since positive results are also found in those who have had B.C.G. vaccination and in many normal people, but it is useful in helping to classify the different tissue responses in leprosy.

The most serious results of leprosy infection consist in peripheral neuropathy, and its sequelae. The principal mixed nerve trunks of the limbs and face may be severely damaged in their superficial course. The damage is due to cellular reaction to degenerating leprosy bacilli, rather than to the presence of living organisms, and is shown clinically by distal sensory and motor deficits, with resultant mutilations, contractures and muscular atrophy.

Any determinate form of leprosy may undergo an exacerbation, loosely called a 'reaction', which is regarded as caused by obscure variations in the defence mechanism.

Clinical Features. The disease usually becomes manifest insidiously, although occasionally it does so more abruptly. The most common first symptom is a small but persistent area of impaired sensation. In other cases the first noticeable feature may be macules, which are usually hypopigmented and erythematous.

Tuberculoid leprosy is arbitrarily classified into three types, macular, minor and major tuberculoid. The tuberculoid macule has clear-cut definite margins; the surface is smooth and dry and exhibits some loss of sensation, tactile and thermal appreciation being early impaired. Sensory impairment may not be evident in lesions of the face. The macules are often multiple but asymmetrical. Common sites are the lateral aspects of the arms and legs, the buttocks and shoulders. Minor tuberculoid lesions are slightly raised, particularly at the margin. By extension, large areas may be affected. The distribution is similar to that of macular tuberculoid lesions. Some of the superficial cutaneous nerves supplying the affected areas may be enlarged and tender. Major tuberculoid lesions are larger than minor lesions, and more raised; the centre may be atrophic and flattened, while the edges are raised and advancing. These lesions exhibit loss of appreciation to all three superficial sensory stimuli, loss of sweating and, on exposure to cold, lack of contraction of the arrectores pilorum muscles. Related nerve trunks are typically enlarged, hard and tender at sites of predilection.

The main complications of tuberculoid leprosy are the result of accompanying peripheral neuropathy resulting from cellular infiltration, leading to fibrosis and sometimes caseation in the nerves. A combination of fifth and seventh cranial nerve damage produces an exposed anaesthetic eye very liable to loss of sight from trauma and infection. In the upper limbs destruction of the ulnar nerve may lead to a claw hand and ulceration of the phalanges. Evidence of enlargement of the great auricular, ulnar, lateral popliteal or other nerves, is a valuable aid in diagnosis. Osteomyelitis consequent upon infection through an abrasion in an insensitive area may cause the loss of terminal portions of digits, but more commonly the phalanges are absorbed until the finger nails may appear to arise from the knuckles. In the lower limbs foot-drop and traumatic lesions of insensitive feet are very common.

The macule of *indeterminate leprosy* is an inconspicuous lesion 2 to 3 cm. in diameter, situated anywhere on the body, exhibiting slight pigmentary and sensory changes. This lesion often heals spontaneously.

Borderline or *dimorphous leprosy* may present as annular lesions of bizarre shape with ill-defined outer margins, or by plaques and succulent lesions more raised at the centre than at the periphery.

Lepromatous lesions of the skin are described as they progress from early to late lesions, as being macular, infiltrative, diffuse or nodular. Lepromatous macules are numerous, hypopigmented, erythematous, and very slightly infiltrated. They differ from tuberculoid macules in that they are small, widely scattered on the body, usually symmetrically, and the margins of the macules merge imperceptibly with normal skin. Sensation in them is not impaired. They are often inconspicuous except to the trained eye and to local inhabitants who are often familiar with the signs that herald grave leprosy. Although clinically the lesions are not very obvious, the diagnosis is not difficult for *Myco. leprae* are numerous in the skin and can be demonstrated by skin-slit as described below. As the disease advances, the macular lesions become infiltrated and succulent in appearance; in advanced lepromatous leprosy nodular lesions appear, especially on the ears and face. A less common manifestation of lepromatous leprosy is diffuse symmetrical thickening of the skin, often with thickened lobes of the ear, producing 'leonine facies'.

With advanced lepromatous disease 'glove and stocking' peripheral anaesthesia is frequently present, but nerve damage occurs typically later than in the other determinate forms of leprosy. The outer third of the eyebrows is often lost. Impairment of sweating occurs.

The following extradermal lepromatous lesions should be noted. The testes may be destroyed and gynaecomastia ensue. The mucous membranes of the nose, mouth and trachea may ulcerate, and late deformities may result from necrosis of the cartilage and bones of the nose and oral cavity and loss of the upper incisor teeth. The lips and face may be grossly misshapen. Adjacent lesions may spread into the eye but, more commonly, this is infected through the blood stream. The most frequent lesions in the eye are miliary lepromata on the iris and accompanying superficial punctate keratitis, but any part of the eye except the retina may be affected. An acute irido-cyclitis frequently supervenes during the acute exacerbation of lepromatous leprosy.

Reactions. Untreated leprosy does not show a steady progression. Many patients with tuberculoid leprosy overcome the infection with minimal residual signs. Lepromatous leprosy tends to smoulder for a time with gradual progression but, after the disease has become extensive, 'lepra reactions' may ensue. These are characterised by fever, exacerbation of existing lesions and the appearance of new ones and of an eruption aptly called 'erythema nodosum leprosum'. In addition, subcutaneous nodules, iritis, orchitis, lymphadenitis, ulceration of nodules, pain in nerves and oedema of extremities may develop. During the lepra reaction the ESR rises. After the reaction has subsided the disease will be found to have extended. A series of such reactions may lead the patient gradually towards death. In tuberculoid leprosy, too, reactions may occur and these are very liable to be precipitated by large initial doses of dapsone, or over-rapid increments. The reactions consist of exacerbation of existing skin lesions with surrounding oedema and an increase of organisms rendering the patient temporarily infective. Lesions become hypersensitive, while swollen peripheral nerves, constricted at places by the epineurium, may be extremely painful. In summary, pain rather than fever or toxicity is predominant. Reactional states are attributable to inadequate or dis-ordered defence mechanisms. In tuberculoid leprosy it may be an 'up-grading' reaction leading to regression of the disease, but during the reactions damage of importance may be sustained, especially in nerves or the eye, and unstable intermediate forms may exhibit a loss of im-munity progressing towards the lepromatous type. Some reactions, how-ever, are mild, consisting chiefly in swellings of 'erythema nodosum leprosum', each lasting for only a few days and recurring over several months.

Diagnosis. There are many causes for the appearance of macules but a hypopigmented macule with a well-defined edge associated with sensory changes, which cannot be attributed to scarring, is very suggestive of tuberculoid leprosy. If such a lesion is associated with definite enlargement of nerves a clinical diagnosis needs no further confirmation. *Myco. leprae* are unlikely to be demonstrable in the skin but a biopsy taken from the edge of a lesion will show the characteristic histology. A nerve biopsy will demonstrate cellular infiltration and sometimes the organisms, but this is seldom necessary for diagnosis.

Lepromatous leprosy is readily diagnosed by the demonstration of *Myco. leprae* stained by a modified Ziehl-Neelsen's method in material obtained from the deeper layers of the skin on the point of a scalpel introduced through a small slit in the skin. A smear made from a fragment of mucosa obtained from the nasal septum may contain characteristic globi of *Myco. leprae*. The presence of *Myco. leprae* distinguishes lepro-matous leprosy from other diseases of the skin, e.g. diffuse cutaneous leishmaniasis (p. 5).

There are very few conditions other than leprosy that give rise to enlargement of nerves. Local enlargement may be due to a neuroma or trauma. Wasting may make nerves more easily palpable than normally; hence, asymmetrical enlargement is of particular clinical significance. Enlargement of one or more nerves may occur in primary amyloidosis. Familial hypertrophic neuritis is a rare familial disorder. An over-anxious wearer of a bush-shirt who rests his elbows on a desk may need reassurance that his palpable ulnar nerves are not pathologically thickened. Usually the polyneuritis of leprosy is associated with cutaneous lesions but in some countries pure 'neural forms' are not uncommon. Syringomyelia may be simulated, but the sensation of touch is lost early in leprosy and

B

retained in syringomyelia, which may also be associated with upper motor neurone lesions in the lower limbs.

Treatment. To enable specific treatment to be carried out successfully it is important to win the confidence and collaboration of the patient. Multiplication of *Myco. leprae* is inhibited by dapsone (diamino-diphenyl-sulphone, DDS) taken orally. Clinical observations and recent experimental work indicate that only very small doses are required, although the emergence of organisms showing resistance to dapsone indicates that there may be a danger in using minimally effective doses. Toxic effects of the drug and precipitation of reactional states are much less likely to occur, however, if small doses are employed. It will usually be appropriate to administer 25 mg. weekly, increasing this by 25 mg. weekly, until a dose of 50 mg. twice weekly is reached. For lepromatous leprosy double this dose may be required. For children under 5 years, one-fifth of the adult dose, and from 5 to 12 years one-half of the adult dose should be prescribed.

In tuberculoid leprosy the tendency is towards arrest, but cure may be hastened and deformity prevented by early treatment with dapsone. This should be continued for a minimum of 2 years and for not less than 12 months after apparent cure. Patients with borderline leprosy require careful supervision and cautious treatment. The clinical manifestations of lepromatous leprosy may be dramatically affected or response may be extremely slow, but in any case treatment must be continued for at least 2 years after skin smears are negative. The patient must be prepared to accept treatment lasting for many years and perhaps for life. Follow-up is essential as relapses have been reported, especially in patients with borderline leprosy, inadequately treated.

The proportion of the normal to the degenerate bacilli is called the morphological index, which is one indication of the bacteriostatic activity of the drug used, and hence a criterion for eventual clinical improvement. Morphologically normal bacilli ('solid rods') usually disappear in a few months from the sites from which smears are taken, and such patients may thereafter be considered to be non-contagious.

Toxic effects, which are largely avoided by the above cautious regime, include anaemia, dermatitis, erythema nodosum leprosum, neuritis, hepatitis and psychosis. Pain due to swelling of the nerve may be distressing and may be followed by increased neural damage (see below).

Thiambutosine is a satisfactory substitute for dapsone. The dose is 500 mg. (1 tablet) daily for a fortnight increasing by 500 mg. fortnightly to a maximum of 2 to 3 g. daily. It is less liable to cause toxic effects than dapsone but drug resistance may occur after two years of treatment with it.

Some long-acting sulphonamides (e.g. sulfadoxine) are widely used in some countries.

Patients who do not tolerate dapsone may be treated with considerable success by a combination of isoniazid and streptomycin which is also indicated if there is concomitant tuberculosis. Rifampicin, of proved value in the treatment of tuberculosis, has recently been used successfully in leprosy. Clofazimine (Lamprene) is particularly indicated in the treatment of reactional states (see below).

Those with areas of anaesthesia (thermal and tactile) must be given careful instructions regarding measures to prevent damage to the affected part. Physiotherapy should be started early in the disease. Orthopaedic measures are often necessary to correct deformities resulting from damaged peripheral nerves. Thus ideally every patient with neural damage should be early subject to orthopaedic control.

TREATMENT OF REACTIONS IN LEPROSY. If the patient is suffering from hepatitis, a psychosis or an allergic dermatosis attributable to dapsone, this drug should be stopped. In other cases of active leprosy in which the dose of dapsone has not been too high, it or an alternative anti-leprosy drug should be continued.

Clofazimine (Lamprene, B663) is valuable in that it exerts an anti-inflammatory effect and is at the same time bacteriostatic. It does, however, produce a ruddy complexion and tends to cause dark pigmentation in areas of skin already affected by leprosy. This may make the drug unacceptable to some, but the relief obtained may outweigh the disadvantages. A dose of 100 mg. three times daily will usually suffice to control a reaction. When clofazimine is used, it is seldom necessary to incise the epineurium of swollen nerves or to inject hydrocortisone into the sheath.

For patients in whom clofazimine cannot be given, older methods should be attempted. Chloroquine 150 mg. (base) three times daily for two weeks or, if there is no response, a trivalent antimonial, such as Stibophen, 2 ml. intramuscularly on alternate days for six doses should be tried.

In severe reactions, if clofazimine is declined or fails, corticosteroids, e.g. prednisolone 25 mg. daily, will usually give relief, but there is great difficulty in withdrawing the corticosteroid without risking a rebound exacerbation. If dapsone has been stopped, thiambutosine may be substituted temporarily.

Iridocyclitis, associated with erythema nodosum leprosum, must be treated by dilating the pupils with 1 per cent. atropine drops morning and evening, while hydrocortisone eye drops (1 per cent. solution) are applied hourly until the inflammation subsides. If the patient is not having systemic corticosteroids 5 to 8 mg. of hydrocortisone dissolved in 0·3 ml. sterile normal saline may be injected subconjunctivally. When there is an open corneal ulcer corticosteroids should be given cautiously and then only with an antibiotic.

GENERAL MANAGEMENT. In Britain the disease is notifiable. Voluntary segregation is rarely indicated for lepromatous patients before treatment is established although initiation of treatment in an institution is often beneficial. Good food, regular exercise and efficient treatment of inter-current diseases such as tuberculosis, dysentery, malaria, kala azar and helminthic infections are important. The morale of patients should be maintained by providing social amenities, schools, vocational training and, where possible, agreeable and remunerative occupation.

Personal Prophylaxis. Children should not come into close or repeated contact with open leprosy. Medical staff should take the ordinary pre-cautions of washing of hands with soap and water and wear rubber gloves and gowns when engaged in activities necessitating prolonged contact with the skins of patients with lepromatous leprosy. Dapsone prophylaxis is generally neither necessary nor desirable but a child who has been in close contact with a lepromatous parent may be given oral dapsone for two years after exposure has ceased. Since there is some evidence that B.C.G. vaccination may protect about three-quarters of children exposed intrafamilialy to leprosy, B.C.G. vaccination should be offered to child contacts of patients with lepromatous leprosy. However, the reduction of the reservoir of infection by mass treatment, concentrating on patients with lepromatous and borderline leprosy, appears to offer at present the best prospect of control of the disease in the community.

CHOLERA

Cholera, an acute disease of the gastrointestinal tract, is caused by the contamination of food or drink by strains of *Vibrio cholerae*. There are different strains named Inaba, Ogawa, Hikojima and also *Vibrio eltor*, which since 1961 has become widespread throughout the Far and Near East and appears to be displacing the classical *V. cholerae* from some areas. There have recently been outbreaks also in Africa. Formerly thought to be of low pathogenicity, its virulence is now found to be equal to that of other strains. These disease-producing vibrios have to be distinguished from the many non-pathogenic cholera-like vibrios. The most important endemic foci of cholera are in the lower reaches of the Ganges and Brahmaputra rivers. In these areas epidemics of cholera are likely during the hot moist season when large numbers of people, such as pilgrims, congregate and live in overcrowded and unhygienic conditions, and the disease may spread widely when people incubating it return to their scattered homes. *Vibrio cholerae* usually disappear from the stools of patients within a week of convalescence but exceptionally they may persist up to a month after the acute attack and *V. eltor* may continue to be excreted for as long as three years. There are no chronic carriers.

The disease appears to be maintained in endemic areas by very mild infections in a population with a considerable resistance to it.

Pathology. Apart from the shrinkage of organs and tissues through intense dehydration there is acute diffuse enteritis principally in the small bowel. The capillaries in the intestinal villi are widely dilated; the mucosa, pinkish and coated with mucus, is infiltrated by lymphocytes and the submucosa is often oedematous. The great loss of fluid and electrolytes from the bowel and massive outpouring of hepatic and pancreatic secretions cause intense dehydration, haemoconcentration and acute renal failure. Cholera vibrios do not invade the blood stream but are found only within the superficial layers of the intestinal wall and in its dejecta. Investigations indicate that the local changes in the mucosa of the small intestine are caused by cholera exotoxins which inactivate the mechanism underlying sodium and water absorption and that the vibrio endotoxins on absorption aggravate the hypotensive state brought about by loss of body fluids.

Clinical Features. After an incubation period of a few hours to five days severe diarrhoea without pain or colic, followed by vomiting, usually begins suddenly. This is characteristically effortless, fluid gushing from the bowel and from the stomach. After the faecal contents of the gut have been evacuated the typical 'rice-water' material is passed. This consists of flakes of mucus floating in water. In severely ill patients, which includes most cases of cholera, an enormous quantity of fluid and electrolytes is rapidly lost. This soon leads to intense dehydration with agonising muscular cramps. Soon the patient passes into the 'algid stage' with a low surface temperature, although the rectal temperature may be up to 39° C. (102° F.). Cardiovascular collapse and prostration then accompany a very low blood pressure and a pulse which is barely perceptible; the urine output is very scanty or absent. The body surface is cold and clammy, the eyes sunken and the skin wrinkled. The patient, however, usually remains mentally clear. Unless fluid and electrolytes are replaced early and in adequate amounts the patient may die from acute circulatory failure within 24 hours of the onset of the disease. With proper treatment, however, improvement can be expected, the diarrhoea and vomiting cease, the pulse and blood pressure improve, urine output increases and the 'stage of reaction' sets in. During this stage the patient may develop hyperpyrexia or, if the fluid has not been replaced in time, complete suppression of urine may lead to death from uraemia.

Although this is the typical picture of cholera, other rare types of the disease may be encountered varying from a mild illness with only slight diarrhoea—'ambulant cholera'—to a very intense illness—'cholera sicca'—in which the patient is overwhelmed by the infection and the rapid loss of fluid into the dilated bowel and dies before typical gastrointestinal symptoms appear.

In children under 12 years of age the mortality rate is higher (15 to 17 per cent.) than that of adults (4 to 6 per cent.). Pulmonary oedema, febrile reactions to therapy, pyrexial convulsions and encephalopathy, tetany, meteorism, hypoglycaemia, hypernatraemia, acidosis and water retention and frequently malnutrition are believed to be the adverse factors in paediatric practice. Overhydration and respiratory complications, more common than in adults, may also play a part. Consideration of such factors and of the delicate physiological and biochemical balance in children have led to modifications in their management and treatment (p. 29). These methods have lowered the mortality to slightly below the adult level of 4 per cent.

Diagnosis. During a cholera epidemic the diagnosis is usually easy. It is, however, important that an atypical case should be recognised early so that the outbreak may be brought rapidly under control. Microscopic examination of the stool will detect the typical cholera vibrio, and culture of the stool or a rectal swab on special media is used to isolate the organism and determine its serological characteristics. Other diseases such as acute bacillary dysentery, viral enteritis, *P. falciparum* malaria, food poisoning and certain chemical poisons may produce symptoms like those of cholera. Cholera is notifiable under the International Sanitary Regulations.

Treatment. Three days treatment with tetracycline 250 mg. six-hourly or furazolidine in single daily doses of 400 mg. is of limited value in expediting the disappearance of the vibrios from the stools. The chief aim in treatment, however, is to maintain the circulation and prevent acute renal failure. This can be achieved by replacement of the great loss of water and electrolytes; the earlier this is started, the better is the prognosis. A clinical assessment of the patient's need in terms of water and electrolytes can be made from the appearance of the patient, the pulse, blood pressure, the output of urine and from information regarding the volume of fluid lost by diarrhoea and vomiting. Severe depletion of water and salt is usually rapid and this causes dangerous dehydration.

In adults replacement should be provided by intravenous isotonic saline, and in severe dehydration a total of 20 litres or more may be required to make good the loss. In such cases as much as 2 litres, by the intravenous route, may be given in the first hour and 1 litre in the second and in the third hours. As the veins are contracted it is usually necessary to introduce a cannula or preferably a polythene tube into a large vein. Subsequent fluid is given as indicated by the condition of the patient, a careful watch being kept for signs of pulmonary oedema and on the urinary output.

To counteract acidosis it is necessary during hydration to give 1 litre of isotonic (18·7 g. per litre) sodium lactate solution for every 2 litres of isotonic saline. If modern facilities exist for the correct sterilisation and storage of isotonic sodium bicarbonate solution (14 g. per litre), this solution is now considered preferable to sodium lactate solution (p. 232), as with the latter lactic acid acidosis may develop in conditions of shock. Should hyperpyrexia occur, corticosteroids may help to control it, and they may also be of value for a severely shocked patient.

The rectal temperature, and fluid loss in vomit and stool, and output of urine should be carefully recorded. Stools should be collected in a calibrated plastic receptacle under a 'cholera cot' which has a central reinforced hole and funnel, over which the patient's buttocks are placed. When there is doubt about the need for further fluid, an estimation is made of the patient's whole blood specific gravity using the copper sulphate drop method. A rise in specific gravity of 0·001 above the normal 1·055 indicates a lack of approximately 150 ml. of fluid in a man weighing about 70 kg. Once vomiting has ceased, as much fluid as possible should be taken by mouth. Fluids given by an intragastric drip may successfully reduce the quantity of intravenous fluid required.

It is safer not to replace potassium loss until the kidneys have started to function freely. Then potassium citrate 2 to 4 g. should be given three times a day by mouth or 10 m.Eq (0·75 g.) potassium chloride can be added to each litre of the intravenous fluid. In Pakistan good results have been obtained by the intravenous infusion of an aqueous solution containing in each litre sodium chloride 5 g., sodium bicarbonate 4 g., potassium chloride 1 g. The 'milk' of green coconuts is a useful source of potassium for oral administration. Anuria makes the prognosis very grave. Treatment should be given for it as recommended on page 725. Favourable results from the use of corticosteroids have been reported in a limited number of cases of cholera.

In children quick initial hydration is required but after the critical stage has passed overhydration, failure of correction of acidosis or a sudden swing to alkalosis may produce a fatal result. Therefore, although the principles remain the same as in adult therapy, certain modifications are required. Calculation of fluid requirements on the basis of the specific gravity of whole blood or plasma are excessive for a child of body weight less than 15 kg. Limb veins are extremely difficult to find in the collapsed child, therefore a scalp vein or the external jugular vein should be selected for infusion. Intraperitoneal infusion has been found effective in the very young, but cholera is relatively uncommon below the age of 6 months. Ringer lactate (B.P.) with pH adjusted to 7 is the fluid of choice and is given at a rate of 30 ml./kg. body weight in the first hour, but this may be varied according to the severity of dehydration and is thereafter regulated to replace the fluid loss in vomit, stool and urine. Glucose water by mouth is given as soon as tolerated. Tetany, convulsions and hypogly-caemia may also require treatment.

Once convalescence sets in it is rapid and uneventful.

Personal Prophylaxis. All discharges and soiled articles of clothing must be disinfected. Gloves should be worn by nursing attendants. Drinking water should be boiled, all food cooked and both protected from flies. Vaccination with a killed suspension of *V. cholerae* should be given in two doses, 0·5 and 1·0 ml. with an interval of one to four weeks. It is an international requirement for travellers passing through endemic zones to be in possession of a certificate of vaccination which becomes valid six days after the first dose and lasts for six months. A controlled trial has shown that the vaccines in current use only reduce the expected incidence of cholera by 26 per cent. but combined with an aware-ness for the need for improved hygiene may lead to the abrupt cessation of an outbreak.

Some cholera vaccines produce cross-agglutination with brucellae, and this may subsequently confuse investigations of a fever.

ANTHRAX

For centuries anthrax has been known as a disease of domestic animals. They become infected by inhaling or ingesting spores. The *Bacillus anthracis* passed in faeces forms spores in the presence of oxygen which become widely disseminated by air currents. Grazing lands remain infective for years and it is necessary to bury infected carcasses deeply to avoid contamination of the soil.

In man it is an occupational disease of farmers, butchers and dealers in hides, animal hair and wool and handlers of bone meal from endemic areas. In primitive conditions, where skins are used as sleeping mats, for clothing or for carrying water, and where diseased cattle are eaten, the infection occurs endemically.

The primary lesion in man may be in the skin, pharynx, larynx, lung or intestinal tract, from any of which sites the infection may spread to lymph nodes and lead to a bacteraemia with demonstrable changes in the spleen, lungs, meninges and brain. The microscopical changes are those of haemorrhagic inflammation with areas of necrosis and interstitial oedema. There is a neutrophil leucocytosis of the blood and infiltration in the tissues without abscess formation.

In animals the disease may run a fulminating course, causing death from asphyxia in a few hours to several days, or be more prolonged with the formation of a carbuncle or a swelling around the neck or shoulders.

In man there is an incubation period ranging from one to three days, or less commonly, up to 10 days. When the infection is acquired from a skin or hide or from handling or slaughtering an animal, a cutaneous lesion indicates the portal of entry. This usually takes the form of a solitary 'malignant pustule' on an exposed part of the body, commonly the face. It begins as an itching papule which enlarges and forms a vesicle filled with serosanguineous fluid surrounded by gross oedema. The lesion is relatively painless and accompanied by enlargement of regional lymph nodes. The vesicle dries up to form a thick black 'eschar' surrounded by blebs. In endemic areas patients may exhibit only slight constitutional symptoms but in non-immune persons the lesion is accompanied by high fever and toxaemia and if the sufferer is not energetically treated an overwhelming bacteraemia may prove fatal within a week or be overcome only after a stormy and more prolonged illness. Occasionally there may be no localised pustule but only oedema.

When infected meat is eaten, an ulcer with much surrounding oedema may be seen in the pharynx or more commonly the infection causes a severe gastroenteritis which frequently terminates fatally. Some people, usually of an older age, escape unscathed after eating infected meat, presumably because of previously acquired immunity.

Those who acquire the infection by inhalation (wool-sorters' disease) may develop an acute laryngitis or a virulent haemorrhagic bronchopneumonia.

Diagnosis. The appearance of a cutaneous lesion and the environmental and occupational history should suggest the diagnosis. A stained smear of fluid taken from the edge of a malignant pustule demonstrates the organism, which may be confirmed in an atypical case by culture and pathogenicity tests in mice, rabbits or guinea-pigs. *B. anthracis* is also recoverable in laryngeal and pulmonary infections. If a group of people who have feasted on an animal which has sickened and died are taken abruptly ill with fulminating gastroenteritis, anthrax should be suspected.

Post-mortem examination is not to be lightly undertaken because of the risk of spreading the infection, but the mere demonstration in the faeces of an organism resembling *B. anthracis* requires cultural confirmation as the non-pathogenic *B. subtilis* is a common inhabitant and is morphologically similar. Suspected animal products can be investigated by the addition of anthrax immune serum to a clear extract of boiled tissues, a precipitate forming within 15 minutes if the tissue is infected.

Treatment. *B. anthracis* is sensitive to most antibiotics. Effective treatment consists in giving penicillin or tetracycline in combination with streptomycin, in full doses, for three to five days. In the presence of urgent symptoms, if an anti-anthrax serum of known potency is available it should be administered intravenously, in a dose not exceeding 50 ml.

Prevention. The disease is controlled in cattle by slaughter and deep burial of the diseased animal, by the administration of prophylactic antiserum to healthy animals at risk and by annual immunisation with attenuated cultures. Imports from endemic areas should be subject to strict control and sterilization. A vaccine is used to protect laboratory workers.

PLAGUE

Plague is caused by *Pasteurella pestis* and is primarily an infection of rodents. The organisms are transmitted between rodents by fleas (*Xenopsylla* spp.) and after the death of a rat an infected flea may leave it and bite man. While feeding, the flea regurgitates the organisms from its proventriculus, blocked by plague bacilli, and thus infects man. In some countries wild rodents are the main hosts and from time to time the infection spreads from them to domestic rats and thence to man. In man the bacteraemia may cause pneumonitis with the expectoration of *P. pestis*. Thus the infection may be spread from man to man by aerosols, the condition then being called 'pneumonic plague'. This condition can also be caused by the accidental inhalation of a laboratory culture or dust containing viable organisms from infected rodents.

Pathology. Rarely a vesicle with surrounding cellulitis is evident at the site of the flea-bite. The more usual initial lesion is acute inflammation in and around the lymph nodes regional to the site of entry of the organisms. The nodes are haemorrhagic and surrounded by oedematous haemorrhagic cellular tissue. *P. pestis* are numerous in and around the infected nodes. This regional lymphadenopathy is the basis of the clinical description 'bubonic plague'.

Signs of a haemorrhagic septicaemia are seen in all fatal cases with subpericardial and meningeal haemorrhages. There may be haemorrhagic foci of consolidation in the lungs, enlargement of lymph nodes and spleen and multiple small necrotic foci in the liver. In some severe cases there may be little or no swelling of regional lymph nodes; these are the cases clinically presenting as 'septicaemic plague'. In deaths from 'pneumonic plague' the signs are those of acute congestion in one or more lobes of the lungs and evidence of generalised haemorrhagic septicaemia. *P. pestis* are numerous in all affected organs.

Clinical Features. The incubation period is short, three to six days, but less in pneumonic plague.

BUBONIC PLAGUE. The most common site of the bubo, made up of the swollen lymph nodes and surrounding tissue, is one groin but, according to the site of the biting by the flea, the bubo may instead be axillary, cervical, epitrochlear or popliteal. The onset is usually sudden with a rigor, high fever, dry skin and severe headache. Soon aching and then also swelling at the site of the affected lymph nodes begin. Some cases are relatively mild but in the majority signs of toxaemia rapidly increase, with a rapid pulse, dilated heart and with mental confusion. The spleen is usually palpable.

SEPTICAEMIC PLAGUE. Those not exhibiting a bubo usually, but not invariably, deteriorate rapidly if not treated. Pneumonia and expectoration of blood-stained sputum containing *P. pestis* may complicate bubonic or septicaemic plague.

PNEUMONIC PLAGUE. The onset is very sudden with cough and dyspnoea. The patient expectorates copious blood-stained frothy, highly infective sputum, becomes cyanosed and rapidly deteriorates. Moist sounds are heard in the lungs but there are no signs indicating consolidation.

Diagnosis. Early diagnosis is urgent. A report of deaths among rats or of human infection should alert all medical personnel. Especially under these circumstances a bubo, with no evident local pyogenic cause for it, must be punctured, using a dry syringe and needle. Staining a smear of the aspirate with methylene blue will show the characteristic bipolar appearance of the organisms. For confirmation the aspirate or blood can be cultured. A leucocytosis distinguishes 'septicaemic plague' from typhoid fever; blood culture is usually necessary to establish the diagnosis although occasionally the organisms can be seen in a stained blood film. The sputum of a patient with pneumonic plague contains very numerous *P. pestis*. Plague is notifiable under the International Sanitary Regulations.

Treatment. Streptomycin is the drug of choice in the treatment of plague. The first dose should be 1 g. intramuscularly, followed by 500 mg. every six hours until the temperature has been normal for 24 hours, after which 1 g. should be given daily for a further six days. Excellent results have been achieved with this course of treatment, especially when it is started early in the disease. Tetracycline has proved to be almost as effective as streptomycin; the initial dose should be given intravenously. The adult oral dose is 1 g. every six hours for 48 hours or longer, depending on the response. After improvement the dose is reduced to 2 g. daily and continued for a further 14 days. In pneumonic or severe septicaemic plague a combination of tetracycline and streptomycin is recommended. If no antibiotic is available, intensive treatment with a sulphonamide should be given. Local treatment of the buboes by the application of glycerine gives considerable relief. The bubo should not be incised unless it points. With antibiotic treatment it is uncommon for suppuration and ulceration to develop.

Personal Prophylaxis. There are two main types of vaccine, the killed vaccine given in two or three doses, and a vaccine containing live avirulent organisms requiring one dose only. The latter has been used with success among indigenous peoples but the killed vaccine is still widely used. Its administration is often followed by a considerable toxic reaction. The immunity conferred is enhanced by revaccination after three to six months. Live avirulent vaccine also usually causes fever, which may last for 5 to 10 days.

Against bubonic and septicaemic plague prophylaxis largely depends on preventing infection by fleas carrying plague. This can be achieved in the case of the domestic rat by preventing its access to food and by the use of bait containing a poison such as warfarin (an anticoagulant) or barium carbonate.

Residual insecticides have revolutionised anti-flea measures. Dusting with insecticides and immunisation by vaccine afford good protection. Powders containing 1·5 per cent. Dieldrin or 2 per cent. Aldrin applied to floors and blown into rat holes kill all the fleas and remain active for 9 to 12 weeks. The insecticide chosen should be one to which the local fleas are known to be susceptible. Contacts should be protected by tetracycline or by intramuscular streptomycin, 1 g. daily for a week, or if this is not available, a sulphonamide such as sulphadimidine 3 to 6 g. daily for the same period. Those attending on patients with pneumonic plague should in addition wear masks, protective gowns and gloves.

TULARAEMIA

Tularaemia is an infection due to *Pasteurella tularensis* transmitted to mammals and birds by the bites of infected blood-sucking flies and ticks. Man may be accidentally infected in a laboratory or while skinning infected wild rabbits or hares. In Norway lemmings are another source. The micro-organisms enter through dermal abrasions, the conjunctiva or mouth. Contaminated water, infected meat and the bites of infected arthropods may also convey the infection to man.

Geographical Distribution. The disease is found in the United States, Canada, Mexico, Japan, Russia, Scandinavia and most European countries.

Pathology. Focal areas of necrosis occur especially in lymph nodes, spleen, liver, kidneys and lungs. There may be cutaneous, oral or ophthalmic lesions when infection is by these routes.

Clinical Features. The incubation period is from 1 to 10 days. There is a sudden onset of high fever followed by sweating and prostration. After some early remission of the fever, the temperature rises again after a few days and remains elevated for 10 to 15 days but in severe infections there may be no early remission and the fever may last continuously for three or four weeks. There is a moderate neutrophil leucocytosis. The spleen is sometimes palpable. About two days after the onset a primary lesion develops in the conjunctiva of one eye or in the skin at the site of an abrasion if the organisms have entered in this way. Such a site is swollen and painful and accompanied by swelling of the regional lymph nodes. When the mouth has been the portal of entry a buccal ulcer or inflamed tonsils may be found. Pleuropulmonary and pericardial inflammatory lesions result from inhalation of the organisms or from haematogenous spread. Lymph nodes may remain enlarged for months.

Diagnosis. The organism may be cultured from the blood although often only after repeated attempts. Guinea-pig inoculation may succeed. An intradermal test using killed *P. tularensis* may be positive as early as the third day, followed by positive agglutination and complement-fixation tests after 10 to 12 days. Antibodies produced by brucellae may also agglutinate suspensions of *P. tularensis*.

Treatment. Most cases respond rapidly to intramuscular streptomycin 2 g. daily. In severe cases the drug should be continued for two weeks. The organism is usually also sensitive to tetracycline.

Prevention. Masks should be worn in the laboratory and gloves should be used when skinning rabbits and hares in endemic areas. Adequate cooking renders infected meat safe for eating.

CHANCROID
(Soft Sore)

This is an important and common venereal disease of the tropics, presenting usually in males since the condition in females is asymptomatic, and difficult to recognise. The causative organism, *Haemophilus ducreyi*, a Gram-negative bacillus, is 1 to 2 microns in length and is seen in pairs, chains or arranged as fish swimming together. Invasion of the lesions by pyogenic organisms is common.

Clinical Features. The incubation period is two to three days, but may occasionally be longer. The initial lesion is a small red papule on the mucous or skin surfaces of the genitalia or on the surrounding skin. In a few days painful necrosis, ulceration and purulent discharge appear, and a well-demarcated surrounding zone of erythema develops. Frequently the lesions are multiple from auto-inoculation and are seen in all stages of development. The inguinal lymph nodes may enlarge, soften and suppurate. General malaise and fever may accompany the local signs.

Diagnosis. Differentiation is required from syphilis, lympho-granuloma inguinale, granuloma venereum and genital herpes. Scraping or aspiration of material from the lesion may reveal the *Haemophilus* which is, however, often overgrown by secondary invaders. Aspiration of a bubo may be more successful. Auto-inoculation of fluid from the lesion on the scarified forearm produces a swelling in which biopsy will demonstrate a recognisable histology. A skin test using a commercial vaccine (e.g. Dmelcos) is also available. Opinions vary as to the value of the two latter tests.

Treatment. It is vital not to mask or miss associated syphilis; therefore only local cleansing with saline should be undertaken and an oral sulphonamide administered until four dark-ground examinations have failed to reveal *Treponema pallidum*. Thereafter excellent results will be obtained with tetracycline, streptomycin or chloramphenicol. Serological tests to exclude latent syphilis should be carried out three months after the completion of the course of treatment.

YAWS
(Framboesia)

Yaws is a disease of certain underdeveloped tropical countries where it is to be found among the more backward indigenous people remote from progressive influences. The cause is *Treponema pertenue*, morphologically indistinguishable from the causative organisms of syphilis and pinta. Serological changes are almost identical with those produced by syphilis. Organisms are transmitted by bodily contact from a patient with infectious yaws through minor abrasions of the skin of another person, usually a child. Infection is most likely to take place in huts at night when the temperature and humidity are high and families use communal sleeping mats.

Geographical Distribution. Areas of infection exist in Mexico, Panama, the Northern parts of South America, West Indies, Central, East and West Africa, the Pacific Islands, Malaysia, Burma, Thailand (uncommonly in India and Ceylon), and also in Indonesia and the Far East, including China where it extends into temperate zones.

Pathology. At the site of the inoculation a proliferative granuloma develops containing numerous treponemata. This primary lesion is followed by eruptions, the most characteristic being multiple papillomatous lesions of the skin with a histology similar to the primary lesion. In addition there may be hypertrophic periosteal lesions of many bones with underlying cortical rarefaction. All these lesions of 'early yaws' heal without appreciable scarring or deformity unless there has been secondary infection. After a variable interval 'late yaws' may develop, characterised by destructive lesions which closely resemble the gummata of tertiary syphilis and which on healing produce much scarring and deformity.

Clinical Features. The incubation period is three to four weeks. The primary lesion or 'mother yaw' is usually on the leg or buttocks and may arise at the site of contact when a child is carried by an infectious adult. The secondary eruption usually follows a few weeks or months later, sometimes before the primary lesion has healed. The most typical are the so-called papillomata, often very numerous, consisting of exuberant tissue covered with a whitish-yellow exudate, and more prolific in the moist flexures and around the mouth. There may be successive crops of lesions. In spite of an eruption of a formidable appearance, the subject, usually a child, is not in a toxic state but may be active and relatively unconcerned except for the irritation caused by the sores and the attentions of the flies which they attract. These lesions are highly contagious. Sometimes a pathologically similar lesion erupts through the palm or sole, when walking becomes painful. The resultant gait has given rise to the description, 'wet crab yaws' which may also be produced by more diffuse hyperkeratotic lesions with cracks in the skin. The bones of all the fingers distal to the carpus, except the terminal phalanges, particularly in children, may rarify and be surrounded by periosteal deposits. The swollen fingers are then aptly described as resembling sausages. There may be a similar swelling of a long bone and also of the nasal bone (goundou). The distorted tibia may remain as the sabre tibia but most of the lesions of early yaws will eventually subside almost completely and spontaneously. Healing is much more rapid after the administration of penicillin. Other lesions of early yaws include a variety of cutaneous eruptions, synovitis and diffuse ganglia.

LATENT YAWS. Following the spontaneous resolution of early yaws serological changes may persist, to be followed by further manifestations of 'early yaws' or, after an interval of as much as 5 to 10 years, by the tertiary lesions of 'late yaws'.

LATE YAWS. Solitary or multiple nodular lesions may develop. They soon ulcerate and spread superficially and also, in places, penetrate deeply into the underlying tissue. In this way gross disfigurement may be caused with distressing ulceration and deformity. There is some evidence that the site of development of late yaws may be influenced by sensitivity to local reinfection with treponemata. Thus a mother with latent yaws, nursing a child with early yaws of the face, may develop a tertiary ulcer on the breast. The lesions of late yaws tend to heal with scarring in one part even while the ulcer is extending in another direction. In addition, in radiographs, localised areas of rarefaction may be shown in long bones with surrounding periostitis. Clinically these present as localised swellings of bones and the overlying tissue may ulcerate giving a picture resembling the gummatous ulceration of tertiary syphilis. Lesions of a solitary bone in the hand may lead to the destruction of the bone and deformity. Lesions of the scalp and underlying localised osteitis of the outer table of the skull are common. The bones of the nose and palate may share in this process. Minor degrees of a sunken nasal bridge or palatal perforation are common and gross mutilation making the nose and mouth one open cavity (gangosa) is one of the most tragic results still compatible with life. The plight of other untreated patients may also be very pitiful, with distortion of bones, contraction of joints, ulceration and scarring. Other late lesions include hyperkeratosis with fissuring of the palms and soles (dry crab yaws), hydrarthrosis, bursitis and juxta-articular nodules consisting of painless, firm, subcutaneous fibrous deposits about the elbows, hips and knees.

Unlike tertiary syphilis, yaws does not affect the cardiovascular system or internal viscera, and the only neurological changes are very minor alterations of the cerebrospinal fluid.

Treatment. Long-acting penicillin is highly effective. Very good results follow the intramuscular administration of 1·2 mega units of PAM (procaine benzylpenicillin with 2 per cent. aluminium monostearate) on two occasions with an interval of one week. For a mass campaign a single dose of 1·2 mega units is given to all active adult cases and 0·6 mega units to latent cases and contacts, which in areas of high endemicity include the whole of the remainder of the population. Proportionate doses are given to children. A second survey and campaign of treatment should follow within a year to detect and treat relapses and missed cases. Tetracycline 1 to 2 g. daily for five days is as successful as penicillin, but the cost and technical difficulties of ensuring that the drug is taken daily make it suitable only for the treatment of an individual patient who is under proper control.

Prevention. With improved housing and increased cleanliness the disease disappears. Anti-yaws campaigns with antibiotics should therefore be only part of a co-ordinated plan to improve the economy, education and hygienic conditions of the people. In few fields of medicine have chemotherapy and improved hygiene achieved such dramatic success as in yaws.

ENDEMIC (NON-VENEREAL) SYPHILIS (BEJEL).

Sporadic venereal syphilis is usually transmitted by sexual intercourse. In certain tropical countries, where lack of hygiene prevails, a treponematosis occurs as a family disease, the lesions of which show a close resemblance to those of venereal syphilis. This condition has been given the local names of *bejel* in Arabia, *njovera* in Rhodesia, *dichuchwa* in Botswana, *siti* in Gambia and *skerljevo* in Bosnia and was known as *sivvens* or *sibbens* when formerly it was endemic in Scotland. The causative organisms are regarded as modified strains of *Treponema pallidum*, with which they are morphologically identical. The Johns Hopkins International Treponematosis Laboratory has reported strains from patients with endemic syphilis as exhibiting in the laboratory constant biological differences from *T. pallidum* obtained from venereal syphilis and from *T. pertenue* and *T. carateum*, the causes of yaws and pinta respectively.

Congenital infections are extremely rare and it is unusual for the infection to be acquired by sexual intercourse. The common mode of infection is through an abrasion, the disease being transmitted from one child to another and occasionally from a child to a parent. Sometimes it spreads in a closed community by the use of common drinking vessels and possibly, on occasions, mechanically by flies. The poor social conditions in which the disease prevails are similar to those where yaws is found but the clinical lesions resemble those of juvenile syphilis.

In contrast to sporadic venereal syphilis the primary lesion is rarely seen, except when a child has inoculated the nipple of the mother during suckling. The lesion presents as an ulcerative papule without regional adenitis. The secondary and tertiary lesions include all the common types of skin and bone manifestations of syphilis but typical papillomatous lesions resembling yaws are infrequent. In addition, 'mucous patches', due to superficial ulceration, in the mouth are common and are often the first sign of endemic syphilis but they are very rare in yaws. Visceral and neurological lesions are absent or rare. The usual serological tests give identical results in sporadic syphilis, endemic syphilis and yaws.

Treatment. The disease responds to treatment by penicillin in the same way as sporadic syphilis. In the social conditions in which it is found the treatment of choice is usually a long-acting penicillin, e.g. PAM (p. 38). Prevention depends on the development of improved social and economic conditions and the mass treatment of affected communities with penicillin.

PINTA

Pinta is an infection caused by *Treponema carateum*, morphologically indistinguishable from *T. pallidum* and *T. pertenue*. It is spread in the same way as non-venereal syphilis.

Geographical Distribution. Pinta is endemic in localised areas in Central and South America and in some West Indian and South Pacific Islands.

Clinical Features. The incubation period is 14 to 20 days. There is a primary scaly papular lesion on an exposed part, usually the leg. The lesion enlarges slowly, up to 10 cm. in diameter and is surrounded by smaller papules. Regional lymph nodes enlarge and like the primary lesion contain treponemata. The second stage is manifest 5 to 12 months later and consists of a generalised eruption of macules and miliary papules (pintids), pinkish and slightly scaly. Most of these heal but others coalesce and form hyperpigmented patches, commonly on the face and exposed parts. The secondary lesions may persist for years and may be accompanied by hyperkeratosis of palms and soles. In the tertiary stage the affected patches become atrophic and depigmented and in some cases extensive white areas result (vitiligo). In the second and tertiary stages there are serological changes closely resembling those of syphilis but pinta does not protect against syphilis, nor syphilis against pinta. Treatment is by a long-acting penicillin, e.g. PAM (p. 38).

THE RELAPSING FEVERS

The relapsing fevers are a group of diseases due to infections by spirochaetes of the genus *Borrelia* transmitted by lice or soft ticks. The louse-borne *Borrelia recurrentis* infects only man and is not transmitted from a louse to its progeny. This disease appears in epidemics when man is living in conditions under which infestation with the human body-louse, *Pediculus humanus corporis*, is frequent and an infected louse is introduced. It may accompany louse-borne typhus fever. The disease is endemic in Ethiopia from where recently recorded epidemics have probably arisen. Epidemics occur in the tropics as well as in cold climates.

Bor. duttoni, the cause of tick-borne relapsing fever, is transmitted by various species of the genus *Ornithodorus*. These ticks may survive for years even under unfavourable conditions. Once a tick becomes infected, it not only remains infected for life but it conveys the infection to its offspring. Tick-borne relapsing fever is thus an endemic disease. The different species of borrelia are morphologically identical.

Louse-borne Relapsing Fever

The borreliae are liberated from the louse when it is crushed during scratching and the same action, prompted by the irritation of repeated bites from lice, inoculates the borreliae into the skin through excoriations.

Pathology. The borreliae live in the blood, where they are abundant in the febrile phases, and invade the liver, spleen and meninges. Hepatitis causing jaundice is frequent in severe infections and there may be petechial haemorrhages in the skin, mucous membranes and serous surfaces of internal organs.

CLINICAL PATHOLOGY. A neutrophil leucocytosis accompanies the febrile period but is replaced by leucopenia in the apyrexial intervals. In the pyrexial phases borreliae are demonstrable in the blood between the erythrocytes. Thrombocytopenia is marked and impaired liver function tests commonly occur. The urine frequently contains protein and sometimes there is frank haematuria. The cerebrospinal fluid is often under raised pressure with an increase of mononuclear cells; sometimes in severe infections pus cells and borreliae may be demonstrable in the centrifuged deposit.

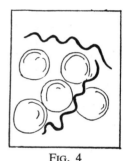

FIG. 4

Borreliae in blood film.

Clinical Features. After an incubation period varying from 2 to 12 days there is a sudden onset of fever. The temperature rises to 39·5° to 40·5° C. (103° to 105° F.) and is accompanied by a rapid pulse, headache, generalised aching, injected conjunctivae and frequently epistaxis and herpes labialis. As the disease progresses, the liver and spleen become tender and frequently palpable, jaundice is common and a petechial rash may appear. Mental confusion and meningism may occur. The fever ends by crisis between the fourth and tenth day, often associated with profuse sweating, hypotension and circulatory failure. There may be no further fever but, in a proportion of cases, after an afebrile period of about seven days there is a recurrence which is usually milder and less prolonged. Occasionally this relapse is followed by one or two further bouts of fever. In the absence of specific treatment there is a considerable mortality, especially among the elderly and malnourished.

Diagnosis. The organisms are demonstrated in the blood during fever either by dark ground illumination of a wet film or by staining thick and thin films. Cultural methods may also be used. Louse-borne relapsing fever is notifiable under the International Sanitary Regulations.

Treatment. Tetracycline is effective but may be followed by a Jarisch-Herxheimer reaction. The initial daily dose for an adult should not exceed 1·0 g. in four divided doses. In patients in a precarious state, initial penicillin may prevent a severe reaction to tetracycline. During the apyrexial period 1 g. daily should be given for seven days and after a week's interval this course should be repeated to ensure that there will not be a late relapse.

Personal Protection. The patient and his clothing and all contacts must be freed from lice as in epidemic typhus (p. 67).

Tick-borne Relapsing Fever

This disease, due to *Borrelia duttoni*, is conveyed by a variety of ticks and its endemicity is governed by the presence of the vector. In the Mediterranean area *Ornithodorus tholozani* is responsible; in the Middle East, Persia, Afghanistan and India and in the New World there are other vectors. These ticks can become infected from rodents or bats as well as by congenital transmission and man is only an incidental host. In Central and East Africa, however, *O. moubata* is the vector and man is probably the only important mammalian host. The disease in these areas is thus confined to old camp sites, old houses and their immediate surroundings, infested with *O. moubata* infected from man or by congenital transmission. The *O. moubata* lives in dried mud floors and the cracks of the walls of huts plastered with mud.

Pathology. The changes resemble those of louse-borne relapsing fever but with late neurological lesions.

Clinical Features. These are similar to those of louse-borne relapsing fever. The febrile bouts, although severe, last usually only for three to five days and the apyrexial periods may also be shorter. Relapses are, however, more frequent and may be as numerous as 10. Iritis and neurological complications, including cranial nerve palsies, optic atrophy, localised palsies and spastic paraplegia, may develop during these later relapses.

Diagnosis. The methods used in diagnosis are similar to those for louse-borne relapsing fever. *Bor. duttoni* are, however, scantier in the peripheral blood but laboratory animals are readily infected.

Treatment. This is the same as for louse-borne relapsing fever.

Personal Protection. Ticks can be killed by lindane (gamma BHC) applied to the inside of the walls and across the entrance to houses.

RAT-BITE FEVERS

There are two rat-bite fevers, one caused by *Spirillum minus*, the other by *Streptobacillus moniliformis*. The latter in addition to being transmitted by a rat-bite has also occurred as an epidemic due to infected milk (Haverhill fever) and in other cases also there has been no known contact with rats or mice.

Geographical Distribution. Both infections are worldwide.

Pathological and Clinical Features. The manifestations of both are very similar. In *Sp. minus* infection (Sodoku) the wound usually heals. After 5 to 21 days it suddenly becomes inflamed, indurated, purplish and painful; it may ulcerate and this stage is accompanied by lymphangitis, regional lymphadenitis, leucocytosis, splenomegaly and fever. After a week the local and general reactions subside but recur after a further few days. Periods of fever lasting 24 to 48 hours are followed by a rapid fall of temperature and, without treatment, febrile bouts may continue to recur for weeks and the patient becomes anaemic. A macular or maculopapular dusky red rash, sparse over the trunk and extremities, appears during the febrile phases. In contrast to streptobacillus fever arthritis is not common.

In streptobacillus (Haverhill) fever the incubation period is one to five days. The bite usually heals well but occasionally an abscess forms in the wound. Regional lymphadenopathy is not marked. The general symptoms resemble those of *Sp. minus* infections but there is frequently painful arthritis and it is unusual to have recurrences of fever after the initial bout which only lasts 48 to 72 hours. Sometimes painful swollen joints may be accompanied by a remittent fever suggesting sepsis.

Diagnosis. *Sp. minus* can be demonstrated in the exudate from the inflamed bite or in fluid aspirated from a lymph node, either by examination under dark-ground illumination or by inoculation intraperitoneally into an uninfected mouse. Blood similarly inoculated into mice or guinea-pigs will yield *Sp. minus* in the peritoneal fluid 5 to 14 days later. The serum yields false positive serological tests for syphilis. In *Strep. moniliformis* infections specific seroagglutinins are demonstrable after 10 days. A titre of 1 in 80 or a rising titre is considered diagnostic but the serological tests for syphilis are negative. The organism can be recovered from the blood or, more easily, from an effusion into an inflamed joint, by culture on media containing serum or ascitic fluid or by intraperitoneal inoculation of mice.

Treatment. Both infections are readily cured by the following antibiotics: penicillin, streptomycin and tetracycline.

Diseases due to Viruses and Rickettsiae

DISEASES DUE TO ARBOVIRUSES

In addition to rabies and the cosmopolitan diseases such as poliomyelitis, measles, influenza and smallpox, transmitted by direct contact, faecal contamination, or through the air, there are, in the tropics, a large number of viruses pathogenic to man which are arthropod-borne, now known by the abbreviation 'arboviruses'. The majority give rise to a febrile illness of brief duration, following which there is partial or complete immunity against further attacks. Some, in the non-immune, may on occasions be neurotropic, giving rise to encephalitis of varying severity. Others, notably yellow fever, may show viscerotropic activity, although it is now recognised that many mild cases of yellow fever occur without appreciable impairment of hepatic or renal function.

On recovery from a viral illness immune antibodies are demonstrable in the sera.

Arboviruses are divided on the basis of their antigenic behaviour into groups.

Group A. In this group are included the viruses of Eastern, Western and Venezuelan equine encephalitis; Chikungunya, O'nyong-nyong and Semiliki Forest fevers. All these are conveyed by mosquitoes.

Group B. This group includes the viruses of yellow fever, dengue, Japanese B encephalitis, West Nile, St. Louis and Murray Valley fevers conveyed by mosquitoes, and those of Kyasanur Forest disease, diphasic meningo-encephalitis, Russian spring-summer fever, louping-ill and Omsk haemorrhagic fever, conveyed by ticks.

Group C. This group now comprises a number of viruses limited to South America.

The remaining arboviruses are placed in a number of small groups or are at present ungrouped. Of particular importance are the viruses causing sandfly fever (p. 51). Haemorrhagic fever with renal syndrome (formerly called epidemic haemorrhagic fever) is now known to be conveyed to man by aerosols from infected rodents so can no longer be regarded as an arbovirus (p. 54). Argentine and Bolivian haemorrhagic fevers are similarly acquired.

There are over 60 arboviruses known to affect man. Within each group viruses produce certain antibodies common to other members of the same group. This is of considerable interest as there is evidence that after several attacks by members of the same group there may be protection against the remainder. This phenomenon may contribute to yellow fever being often mild or subclinical among the indigenous people of an endemic area.

Although the clinical manifestations in an endemic area may be sufficiently characteristic for a fairly reliable diagnosis to be made of such diseases as dengue, sandfly fever and Kyasanur Forest disease, a certain diagnosis rests upon the isolation of the virus in the early stage of the disease by inoculation of laboratory animals or fertile eggs, or by the demonstration of a significant increase in titre of antibodies in sera taken during and after the illness. Mouse-protection tests were formerly used for this purpose but haemagglutination inhibition or complement-fixation tests are now employed. Moderate increases or the presence of antibodies in a single specimen are not diagnostic of an individual virus since antibodies may be common to a group of viruses. Thus the presence of antibodies to the viruses for dengue I and II in the sera of forest animals does not necessarily indicate that they are a reservoir of infection, as these antibodies may have been provoked by other viral infections.

The accurate elucidation of an infection requires the assistance of a specialised laboratory to which blood and sera should be sent in a thermos flask packed with ice. The identification of the virus may be a laborious and lengthy procedure but may prove to be of extreme importance, as for example, when the outbreak of Kyasanur Forest disease was differentiated from yellow fever.

Prevention of diseases due to arboviruses at present rests mainly on the control of the vectors, but an efficient vaccine against yellow fever is available. Although the incidence of encephalitis is not great, a composite vaccine to protect against such a catastrophic illness would be a boon but is a far-off prospect. At present there are no drugs which are effective against these viruses, but the clinical features may on occasion be mitigated by good nursing and symptomatic treatment.

The more common diseases due to arboviruses are dealt with in the section which follows.

YELLOW FEVER

The virus of yellow fever, belonging to Group B of the arboviruses, is transmitted to man by the bite of an infected Aedes mosquito. The virus is in man's blood for two days before the onset of fever, for the first four days of the fever and exceptionally for longer. The mosquito becomes infective for man 10 to 20 days after ingesting blood containing the virus and remains infective for its life which may be as long as seven months.

Epidemiology. Yellow fever is a human disease but there is also a reservoir of infection in primates and other forest animals. In urban areas the vector is *Aedes aegypti* and here it is a disease limited to human beings, the virus being conveyed from man to man by this mosquito. *A. aegypti* breeds in small collections of water in the vicinity of human dwellings which are also inhabited by the adult mosquitoes. Urban yellow fever is endemic especially in Western and Central Africa, but the areas where it is a risk are much more extensive, stretching from the Atlantic Coast south of the Sahara to the Red Sea and Indian Ocean, and south to Angola and Zambia. Yellow fever is also endemic in the jungles of Panama and South America with the exception of Uruguay and Chile. In forests the virus is conveyed between monkeys by mosquitoes living among the tree tops. Man becomes infected by felling trees and being bitten by these mosquitoes. In Africa monkeys may raid plantations near to forests and *Aedes simpsoni*, present in these rural areas, may become infected by biting the monkeys which are carrying the virus, and later man may be bitten by these mosquitoes. Life-long immunity is conferred by an attack of the disease and babies born to immune mothers are protected for two to four months. From the rarity of overt disease among indigenous people in endemic areas and from serological studies it appears that many acquire immunity from subclinical infections with this and other related arboviruses (p. 46).

Pathology. The main lesions are found in the liver and kidneys but haemorrhages take place into many organs. If the disease has not been rapidly fatal the tissues will be jaundiced at post-mortem. The liver is often normal in size. Degenerative changes in liver cells are widespread but maximal in the mid-zonal region where fatty degeneration is intense. Usually refractile acidophilic bodies 'Councilman bodies' may be seen, as the result of hyaline degeneration of parenchymal cells. With the high power of the microscope an acidophilic intranuclear mass may be detectable, the 'Torres inclusion body'. In addition to haemorrhages under the capsule, the kidney shows the changes of acute tubular necrosis.

Clinical Features. The incubation period is from three to six days. Leucopenia lasts throughout the illness. A mild attack, which is the usual clinical manifestation of the disease in local inhabitants, consists of a short fever accompanied by proteinuria, with little or no jaundice. In those who have no prior immunity the classical attack falls into three phases, the initial fever, a period of calm and a subsequent period of reaction or intoxication. In very severe attacks the third stage is reached without the brief apyrexial calm interval. Virus activity ceases at the end of the first stage, the pathology and clinical features of the third stage being the result of hepatic and renal dysfunction which are the usual causes of death in yellow fever. The onset of the fever is sudden, sometimes with a rigor. There are severe supraorbital headaches, backache and pains in bones. The face is flushed, the conjunctivae injected and the tongue is coated and the edges are red. These symptoms and signs resemble those of a severe attack of dengue. The patient soon becomes prostrated; vomiting may be pronounced and the vomit may contain bile or altered blood. If vomiting persists the prognosis is grave. There is increasing epigastric pain, mental irritability and photophobia. The fever is highest on the first day and then declines. The pulse rate falls more quickly than the temperature, and bradycardia is marked by the third day. This disproportion between pulse and temperature is very characteristic and is known as Faget's sign. The urine contains protein in increasing quantities and, later, casts appear and the volume of urine decreases. At the end of four days the temperature reaches normal and the second stage, the period of calm, is reached. In mild cases recovery may now take place without further fever. In more serious cases the third stage, the period of intoxication, follows after a few hours, the temperature rising but the pulse still remaining slow. Jaundice becomes pronounced and the liver palpable and tender. The urine contains bilirubin and red cell casts. There is bleeding, sometimes profuse, from gums, nose, stomach, intestine and urinary tract; petechiae, and conjunctival haemorrhages and ecchymoses in the skin may appear. The patient remains mentally clear and anxious until near death, which is only briefly preceded by coma. The pulse rate increases rapidly in the late stages. In fulminating infections the patient dies within a few days of the onset. Death rarely occurs in those who survive for 12 days. In some outbreaks meningo-encephalitis has been a prominent feature. In non-fatal cases convalescence is without incident and there is no residual detectable damage to the kidneys, liver or heart.

Diagnosis. In an endemic area fever, leucopenia and proteinuria with or without jaundice should suggest the possibility of yellow fever. Blood, sent in the early stages to a laboratory equipped to investigate viruses, may yield the virus, and tests on sera taken early and late will show the presence of increasing antibodies (p. 46). These results will only be of value in making a retrospective diagnosis, which may, however, be important on public health grounds. Similarly the establishing of the cause of death by histological examination of the liver may be of the utmost importance. The disease is notifiable under the International Sanitary Regulations.

Differential Diagnosis. Mild cases closely resemble dengue or sandfly fever. Fever with jaundice and proteinuria in the tropics may be due to severe falciparum malaria, to blackwater fever or, if there is a leucocytosis, to leptospirosis or relapsing fever, pyogenic infections such as pneumonia and rarely to an amoebic abscess of the liver. In infective hepatitis there is no leucocytosis but the fever usually subsides as the jaundice appears, there is little, if any, proteinuria and the stools may become the colour of clay.

Treatment. There is no specific antiviral agent. The patient should be nursed under a mosquito net for the first four days of the illness. When vomiting is troublesome dehydration should be corrected by intravenous glucose saline and blood transfusions should be given if blood loss is severe. Acute renal failure should be treated (p. **725**).

Personal Protection. A single vaccination with the 17 D nonpathogenic strain of virus, available at internationally recognised centres, gives full protection for at least 10 years, the period of validity of the vaccination certificate. Ten days after vaccination adequate antibodies are present in the blood and the certificate of vaccination becomes valid. The vaccine does not produce any appreciable side-effects in adults, unless they are allergic to egg protein, when desensitisation may be necessary. There is a slight risk of encephalitis following the vaccination of young children, so, if at all possible, vaccination should not be carried out in infants under nine months of age. Where vaccination against smallpox and vaccination against yellow fever are required within a short time, i.e. 21 days, yellow fever vaccination should precede the smallpox vaccination, as the interval can then be safely reduced to 14 days for adults for a primary vaccination against smallpox and to four days for a revaccination. No ill effects have as yet been observed from vaccination during pregnancy but it may be safer to defer vaccination.

Prevention. Only travellers possessing valid certificates of vaccination against yellow fever are allowed to proceed from an endemic area to 'receptive areas', by which is meant countries free from the disease but in which the potential vectors exist. In this way the disease has not yet entered Asia. As an additional precaution mosquito control of airports should be maintained. The urban disease can be eradicated by the abolition of the breeding places of *Aedes aegypti*, by the use of residual insecticides in houses (p. **1113**), and by mass vaccination in endemic areas. If susceptible mosquitoes are present and the virus persists in animals in adjacent forests there remains a risk of an outbreak of yellow fever among the unvaccinated.

DENGUE

Dengue is caused by a Group B arbovirus (p. 45). Six antigenic variants of the dengue virus have been described. The virus is transmitted to man chiefly by the mosquito *Aedes aegypti*, but other species of this genus are potential vectors of the disease. Man is infective to the vector 18 hours before the temperature rises and for at least three days after the onset of symptoms. The mosquito can transmit the disease 8 to 12 days after feeding on a patient suffering from dengue and remains infective for life.

The disease is a risk in many tropical and subtropical countries, especially in coastal areas. It is most prevalent during the hot season when the mosquitoes are numerous. One attack usually gives immunity for about nine months and after several attacks a considerable degree of permanent immunity is attained. Some cross-immunity exists between dengue and other members of the B group of arboviruses, including the virus of yellow fever (p. 46).

Dengue is not usually a fatal disease but deaths occasionally occur in children with the haemorrhagic type described in South-East Asia.

Clinical Features. The incubation period is usually five to six days. The disease varies considerably in its clinical severity. It may be a sharp illness with marked constitutional symptoms and signs lasting for 7 to 10 days or a milder disease resembling sandfly fever, with a raised temperature for only two or three days. The fever may be preceded by malaise and headache for two days before the acute onset, characterised by considerable pyrexia and intense generalised aches and pains especially severe in the orbital region and around the joints. Painful movement of the eyes, photophobia, conjunctival injection and lachrymation are often features of the disease. Nausea, vomiting and anorexia are associated with prostration, insomnia and depression. In severe cases the temperature may remain elevated for seven to eight days. An afebrile interval lasting 24 to 48 hours may intervene at the end of the third day when symptoms subside temporarily, to be followed, with a recurrence of symptoms, by a further febrile period of a day or two ('saddleback fever'). The pulse rate is often slow compared with the temperature, and bradycardia may continue well into convalescence. Groups of superficial lymph nodes, usually the cervical, may be enlarged, but this is never a marked feature of the disease. Leucopenia is present throughout the illness.

A rash may appear, especially during the second febrile period. It is morbilliform but the colour resembles that of a scarlet fever rash. It usually begins on the dorsum of the hands and feet and spreads up the arms and thighs to the trunk. In some patients the rash may be scanty or absent while in others it is vivid and may be followed by desquamation.

After the temperature has fallen, depression and prostration often persist into convalescence. It is, therefore, advisable after a severe attack for the patient to have at least two weeks' holiday, preferably in a cool climate.

Since 1956 there has been a series of outbreaks of dengue in South-East

Asia, sometimes in association with the Chikungunya virus, in which the disease has been complicated by haemorrhages, with a variable mortality among indigenous children, but reaching 10 per cent. of those ill enough to be admitted to hospital.

Diagnosis. This is usually easy in an endemic area when a patient has the characteristic symptoms and signs of dengue. However, mild cases may resemble other virus diseases such as sandfly fever, while a severe attack may be mistaken for anicteric yellow fever, but the absence of urinary changes will help to differentiate it. Malaria is excluded by a careful examination of the blood. The rash may resemble to some extent that of measles but the distribution and colour are different and the absence of Koplik spots and coryza is helpful. When haemorrhages occur the disease may be confused with other exanthemata having haemorrhagic manifestations, particularly smallpox. There are a number of dengue-like diseases due to other arboviruses (p. 45). The virus can be recovered from the blood or its presence deduced from increasing titres in immunological tests on the sera (p. 46). There appear to be no differences in the viruses of dengue I and II recovered from patients with and without haemorrhagic signs.

Treatment. There is no specific treatment. The severe pains can be relieved by large doses of aspirin, paracetamol or codeine, without risk of causing addiction but methadone may have to be resorted to. Blood transfusions and corticosteroids are indicated in the haemorrhagic varieties.

Personal Prophylaxis. The patient is nursed under a mosquito net. Breeding places of Aedes mosquitoes should be abolished and the adults destroyed by insecticides (p. 1113).

SANDFLY FEVER
(Phlebotomus Fever)

Sandfly fever is caused by a small group of closely related arboviruses (p. 51) transmitted by the sandfly *Phlebotomus papatasii* and by other species of this genus. No animal reservoir is known. Man is infective to the vector for 24 hours before and for 24 hours after the onset of the fever. The sandfly can transmit the disease about seven days after biting an infected person and remains infective for life.

This infection is prevalent in islands in and countries around the Mediterranean and eastwards into India, Burma and China, especially during the hot dry season when the vector is plentiful. Those who have recently arrived in an endemic area are particularly liable to be affected.

Local adults do not suffer from the disease, probably because of immunity acquired by previous infections in childhood. One attack confers immunity for only a few months, so repeated reinfections are necessary to maintain a protective level. There is no cross-immunity between dengue and sandfly fever.

Clinical Features. After an incubation period, usually of three to four days, the onset is sudden with a rapid rise of temperature. The symptoms and signs are very similar to those of dengue (p. 50). The fever, however, is usually of shorter duration, up to three days, and there is no rash. Occasionally there may be a recurrence of fever after an interval of a few days. Depression and prostration usually persist for some time after the fever has subsided.

Diagnosis. It is extremely difficult in the early stages to distinguish sandfly fever clinically from dengue, malaria, influenza and other fevers. In an endemic area the general course of the illness suggests the diagnosis, but a blood film should always be examined to exclude malaria. The virus can be recovered from the blood and serological changes develop (p. 46).

Treatment. This is on the same lines as for dengue.

Personal Protection. As the sandfly breeds in cracks and crevices, it is difficult to eradicate it. However, a campaign using insecticides against adult sandflies can be very effective and this, combined with the use of repellents, gives useful protection. The ordinary mosquito net will not keep out the tiny sandfly, and a net of very fine mesh which would be effective is difficult to tolerate in hot weather. Impregnating a mosquito net with an insecticide will, however, prevent penetration of the net by sandflies. Modern buildings replacing crumbling masonry abolish the breeding places of sandflies.

KYASANUR FOREST DISEASE

The arbovirus of Group B, responsible for this disease, caused a fatal epizootic in monkeys in the Shimogo district of Mysore State. It has been shown by immunological tests to affect about 10 per cent. of the rural human population in that area. The vectors are Ixodid ticks of the genus *Haemaphysalis* increased numbers of which had been introduced by the grazing of cattle in the area. This disease, first encountered in 1957, is of great interest as it was at first feared to be an outbreak of yellow fever in Asia and illustrates how changing pastoral activities may lead to unexpected outbreaks of disease.

The chief pathological lesions are found in the liver and kidneys.

Clinical Features. The disease in man may be mild with only a short febrile attack or it may be a severe illness with fever lasting for over a week with great prostration and generalised pains in muscles. Mucosal surfaces may bleed. Some patients may relapse after 9 to 21 days when fever and signs of meningeal irritation may ensue. Jaundice is often prominent. In fatal cases death is usually due to liver failure.

Treatment. The patient requires careful nursing; no specific treatment is known. A prophylactic vaccine has been prepared.

JAPANESE B ENCEPHALITIS

The virus causing this disease belongs to Group B of the arboviruses and is transmitted to man by the bites of infected culicine mosquitoes which probably have fed on infected animals or birds, notably nestling herons. Pigs and other domestic animals have been shown to be possible sources of infection but act chiefly as amplifiers of the virus brought to them by mosquitoes. The virus is widespread in the Pacific Islands from Japan to Guam, in the Philippines, Taiwan, Borneo, Malaysia and Singapore. In endemic areas, although serological surveys indicate a high incidence of subclinical infection, only sporadic cases may be encountered. Nevertheless, devastating epidemics, with a high mortality rate, have occurred.

Pathology. Inflammatory and degenerative changes are found in the brain from which, in a proportion of cases, the virus has been recovered.

Clinical Features. Many infections are subclinical but overt disease may occur at any age, although children are particularly susceptible and not infrequently die. With the development of encephalitis the patient experiences a very severe headache, fever, often with rigors, and vomiting. The physical signs are those of meningo-encephalitis, namely, neck rigidity, congestion of the optic fundi, imperfectly reacting pupils, muscular twitching and tremors; and, in severe cases, progressive coma, muscular rigidity and cranial nerve palsies. In some cases only signs of meningitis are present. The cerebrospinal fluid is under increased pressure and although there may be no immediate increase of cells and protein in it, this usually develops within a few days. The acute illness may last from a few days to two weeks or longer. Convalescence is prolonged and tedious. Persistent neurological damage is only a feature in children and after prolonged illness in adults. The mortality rate in overt disease varies from 15 to 40 per cent.

Diagnosis. The virus has only rarely been recovered from the blood or cerebrospinal fluid but in fatal cases may sometimes be obtained from the brain. Increasing titres of specific antibodies in the blood is the usual basis for diagnosis.

Treatment. There is no specific treatment and the value of corticosteroids has not yet been established. Skilled nursing and aids for the patient in coma, such as tracheostomy and artificial respiration, may be life-saving.

Prevention. The elimination of breeding places of the vector mosquitoes, the use of larvicides or insecticides, where practicable, should be instituted. There is no effective vaccine or other antiviral agent available.

HAEMORRHAGIC FEVER WITH RENAL SYNDROME

This disease, formerly called epidemic haemorrhagic fever, is attributable to a virus, although confirmation of its successful isolation is still awaited. Outbreaks occurred in Manchuria and Korea and it, or a similar disease, has been reported from Scandinavia and Soviet Russia. There is a close association with small mammals, in particular bank voles, and it has been established that man becomes infected by aerosols without the intervention of an arthropod vector.

Pathology. The main changes arise from increased capillary fragility. Thus there are widespread internal haemorrhages and escape into the tissues of fluid rich in protein. Haemorrhages into the anterior lobe of the pituitary and into the adrenals are common post-mortem findings and in the kidneys acute tubular necrosis is evident.

Clinical Features. The incubation period is from 12 to 16 days. The onset is sudden with a temperature of 39·5° C. (103° F.) or higher, the face flushed and the eyes congested. The patient complains of headache, aching all over the body, thirst, abdominal discomfort, nausea and vomiting. After about five days the temperature falls and the second or toxic stage begins. Haemorrhages now take place into the skin and from mucous membranes. The urine contains red cells, casts and a large amount of protein. There is a danger of oliguria and anuria. With the onset of the second afebrile stage prostration increases and there may be severe hypotension. The leucocyte count, low in the early stages, is now much increased, at first with primitive granulocytes and later with primitive lymphocytes, the picture resembling that of leukaemia. The coagulation and prothrombin times are normal, the platelet count is diminished and there is a prolonged bleeding time. Death may ensue in this stage but in favourable cases the third or convalescent stage begins towards the end of the second week, with a plentiful flow of urine of low specific gravity, free from protein and casts. This polyuria may continue for some months. Full recovery is usual but very slow.

Diagnosis. In an endemic area the diagnosis is suggested by the characteristic clinical signs and the successive changes in the blood. Other diseases to be differentiated include leptospirosis, typhus and relapsing fever, thrombocytopenic purpura, leukaemia, haemorrhagic dengue fever and certain other haemorrhagic virus diseases described in Russia.

Treatment. There is no specific remedy. Rest and careful nursing are essential. Only sufficient fluid should be given to maintain the fluid balance. Hypotension may be corrected by intravenous plasma or the slow intravenous infusion of a 10 per cent. glucose solution in sterile water. Oliguria and anuria are treated as advised for acute renal failure (p. **725**). With prolonged polyuria in convalescence, potassium and sodium losses may require replacement.

KURU

This disease is peculiar to the Fore people, and close neighbours, living in a localised area of the eastern highlands of New Guinea. The underlying pathology is a progressive replacement of nerve cells, chiefly of the cerebellum and mid-brain, by gliosis. The symptoms are those of tremor and ataxia, accompanied by emotional instability, with progressive paralysis invariably resulting in death, usually within two years of the onset. Children of both sexes are equally affected but it has only recently been observed over the age of 40 years in men and is much commoner in adult females than in young men. The age of onset in children, in recent years, has become progressively older, suggesting that no recent transmission of the disease has occurred. An infective agent, behaving like a 'slow virus', has been transmitted by direct inoculation from the brain of a human victim into the brain of chimpanzees. After repeated passages from brain, liver or spleen of affected chimpanzees and one race of inoculated spider monkeys the 'virus' now exhibits a fixed incubation period and produces lesions resembling kuru. Kuru thus closely resembles 'scrapie', a disease of sheep and goats. It has been postulated that kuru may have been transmitted by the former local custom of women and children ingesting human brain in cannibal feasts, in which men by custom did not partake. Cannibalism declined between 1956 and 1963

c

when it ceased. At present this theory seems to fit the observed data better than attributing the disease to a genetic disorder.

No known treatment affects the progressive course of kuru.

LYMPHOGRANULOMA INGUINALE
(Lymphopathia venereum, Climatic bubo)

Lymphogranuloma inguinale is caused by a virus of the *Bedsonia* group immunologically related and similar in size to the psittacosis-ornithosis and trachoma viruses. They are large viruses and are sometimes included in the family of Rickettsiales. The disease is venereal and is widely distributed in the tropics, especially in seaports. The virus can be transmitted to monkeys, guinea-pigs and mice, but not to birds, and this readily distinguishes it from the ornithosis virus.

Pathology. The primary herpetiform lesion is small and very superficial. The virus passes from the primary lesion to the regional lymph nodes and there causes proliferation of monocytes and lymphocytes and giant-cell formation at numerous foci within the nodes. Untreated, these foci necrose to form multiple small abscesses. Associated with these changes there is a marked connective tissue proliferation in and around the lymph nodes which become matted together and adherent to the surrounding structures. When the inguinal nodes are affected the overlying skin is also inflamed by the periadenitis.

Clinical Features. After exposure to infection one to four weeks elapse before the evanescent initial lesion appears. In the male this is usually situated on the prepuce or glans penis and often escapes notice. Ten to fifty days after exposure the adjacent lymph nodes enlarge. In the male in the first stage a single node on one side of the groin is usually affected, but soon other nodes become inflamed and many become matted together. The infection may spread to the other groin and occasionally to the pelvic group of lymph nodes. The affected nodes are tender, and as the disease progresses the large swelling in the inguinal region adheres to the underlying tissues and to the overlying shiny purplish skin. Enlargement of the lymph nodes above and below the unyielding inguinal ligament produces the characteristic 'groove sign'. With rest and treatment lesions may heal. Otherwise necrotic foci will form and their thick glairy contents will eventually be discharged through the skin by numerous small sinuses. After this, healing is very slow and often associated with marked scarring. Months may pass before recovery takes place.

In the female the primary lesion is seldom found. From the vagina or from the rectum of either sex the virus passes to the adjacent lymph nodes in the pelvis, and sinus formation will then damage surrounding structures with extremely serious and disabling results. Fistulae may form between the rectum, vagina and urethra, and ulcerative proctitis may cause stricture of the rectum. In the female obstruction to the lymphatics may lead to elephantiasis of the external genitalia. These complications in the female constitute the condition called 'esthiomene'.

Associated with the adenitis there may be fever, prostration and loss of weight.

Diagnosis. Material for the intradermal 'Frei' test was originally pus aspirated from an inguinal node, but this has been replaced by Lygranum, a viral suspension grown on the yolk-sac of the chick embryo. In a positive case 24 hours after an intradermal injection of 0·1 ml. of Lygranum antigen, a papule exceeding 6 mm. in diameter will develop and usually persist for two to three weeks. The same antigen can be used for the complement-fixation test. Both these tests are positive within two to six weeks of the development of the adenitis and remain positive for a very long time. As this antigen contains a component common to ornithosis and trachoma, this must be taken into account in the interpretation of the result.

Treatment. To encourage resolution rest in bed is important. Many cases respond well to a sulphonamide, 4 g. sulphadimidine daily in divided doses for 14 days being a suitable course.

In those resistant to sulphonamides, tetracycline 2 g. daily for 14 days often gives good results.

The inguinal nodes must not be incised but aspiration, where indicated, may give relief. When extensive sinuses have formed, complete excision of the mass of inguinal nodes may be required.

For the results of serious lesions arising from pelvic adenitis and for rectal stricture surgical aid will be required.

TRACHOMA

Trachoma, recognised since the time of Ancient Greece and Egypt, is a specific communicable keratoconjunctivitis, usually of chronic evolution, caused by an agent belonging to the *Bedsonia* group of atypical viruses, and characterised by follicles, papillary hyperplasia, pannus and, in its later stages, cicatrisation. The infecting micro-organism is named the trachoma and inclusion conjunctivitis (TRIC) agent. Young children are particularly vulnerable to infection. Transmission is usually by contact or from fomites in unhygienic surroundings. Evidence is accumulating that some infections occur during birth from the infected genital passages, TRIC agents of similar serotype having been isolated from the eyes of a baby, the vagina of the mother and the urethra of the father.

Geographical Distribution. The disease is particularly common in the hot dry dusty areas of the subtropics and tropics but is also present in Southern Europe, and among immigrants in Britain. Some hundreds of million people suffer from trachoma. The disease varies markedly in incidence and in severity in different geographical areas.

Pathology. The infection lasts for years and may be latent over long periods. Recrudescence may result from secondary bacterial infection or from re-infection by the agent itself. The conjunctiva of the upper lid is first affected with combined vascularisation and cellular infiltration, pannus, spreading to the upper cornea and later to other areas producing corneal opacity and impairment of vision. Cicatricial deformity of the upper tarsal plate is an early feature. Entropion, trichiasis, ectropion and corneal scarring are late results.

Clinical Features. The onset is usually insidious and infection may not be apparent to the patient. Early symptoms of conjunctival irritation or smarting may be ignored. Watering, stickiness and blepharospasm may be noticed in the eyes of children. In underdeveloped areas, unless discovered on surveys, the condition may not be reported until vision begins to fail.

The ophthalmic appearances are described in 4 stages (WHO):

STAGE I.   Immature follicles are seen on the upper tarsal conjunctiva including the central area and early corneal changes are usually present.

STAGE II.   Well developed mature soft follicles are present with papillary hyperplasia. Pannus and corneal infiltrates extend from the upper limbus.

STAGE III.   Some or all of the signs of stage II exist with scarring developing, usually from necrosis of follicles.

STAGE IV.   The follicles and infiltrates of stage III have been replaced by scar tissue and the disease is no longer infectious although further changes in the scars may follow. The degree of scarring varies from minimal involvement to trichiasis, entropion, corneal opacities and gross impairment of vision.

Trachoma may also present as an acute ophthalmia neonatorum with secondary bacterial infection.

Diagnosis. Differentiation from inclusion conjunctivitis (blenorrhoea) may be clinically impossible, and in some countries no clear separation can be made. The conjunctivitides of adenovirus, herpes virus and Newcastle disease may closely resemble trachoma. Clinically an early ptosis due to deformity of the upper tarsal plate and appreciation of the characteristic follicular conjunctivitis on eversion of the lids may be helpful. Vascularity and cellular infiltration may be seen using the slit lamp before being visible to the naked eye. Intracellular inclusion particles (Halberstaedter-Prowazek bodies) are demonstrated in conjunctival scrapings by iodine or immunofluorescent staining. TRIC agent may be isolated in the developing chick embryo or in cell culture.

Treatment. Improvement of the hygienic state is of first importance. Local ophthalmic ointment or oily drops of 1 per cent. chlortetracycline, tetracycline or erythromycin may be used twice daily for three months. In mass therapy in endemic areas such topical application twice daily for three to six consecutive days each month for six months has given good results. In some cases daily 3 per cent. tetracycline ointment is the method of choice. A systemic sulphonamide, e.g. sulpha-methoxypyridazine 0·5 g. daily for three weeks is a useful addition to treatment. Deformity and scarring of the lids, corneal opacities, ulceration and scarring require surgical treatment, after control of local infection.

Prevention. Personal and family cleanliness should be improved. Proper care of the eyes of newborn and of young children is essential. The finding of a case, particularly in a child, should lead to examination of the whole family. Population surveys should lead to discovery and treatment of asymptomatic infections. Trachoma clinics are required in highly endemic areas.

DISEASES DUE TO RICKETTSIAE

Rickettsiae are small organisms, about 0·5 micron in diameter, and are natural inhabitants of the cells of the intestinal canal of arthropods. Some species parasitise higher mammals and are pathogenic to man. Rickettsiae are intermediate between viruses and bacteria and all require living cells for their multiplication. Infection is usually conveyed to man through the skin from excreta of the arthropods but in some vectors the salivary glands are affected and then bites are a mode of infection. Transovarian infection in arthropods to the next generation occurs except with *R. prowazeki* and *R. mooseri,* the causes respectively of louse and flea-borne typhus. The Weil-Felix reaction, which is the non-specific agglutination by the patient's serum of the strains of organisms Proteus

OX 19 or OXK, helps in the differentiation of the infections. The following table gives the reactions in the human infections:

Name of Disease	Vector	Weil-Felix Reaction	
		OX 19	OXK
Epidemic typhus	Louse	+ + +	negative
Endemic typhus	Flea from rat	+ + +	negative
Rocky Mountain spotted fever . .	Tick	+	negative
Other forms of tick typhus . .	Tick	+	variable
Scrub typhus	Larval mite	negative	+ + +
Q (Query) fever	None or tick	negative	negative
Rickettsialpox	Mite from mouse	negative	negative
Trench fever	Louse	negative	negative

Pathology. Rickettsiae are characteristically parasites of the vascular endothelium, especially of capillaries and other small vessels, producing lesions in the skin, central nervous system, heart, lungs, kidneys and skeletal muscles. Endothelial proliferation, associated with a perivascular reaction (nodules of Fraenkel) may cause thromboses and often small haemorrhages. In epidemic typhus the brain and in scrub typhus the cardiovascular system are particularly attacked. A specific pneumonitis is frequent in scrub typhus.

The rash in epidemic, endemic and scrub typhus is at first central, but in tick typhus it starts peripherally. In Q fever only a sparse rash is occasionally seen. An eschar often shows the site of the bite in tick and scrub typhus and in rickettsialpox, but not in epidemic and endemic typhus or in Q fever.

The common clinical findings in this group of diseases are fever, severe prostration, mental disturbance and often a rash. The diagnosis can be established by the Weil-Felix reaction in epidemic, endemic and scrub typhus and by complement-fixation and agglutination tests using antigen from the specific *Rickettsiae* in all infections. *Rickettsiae* can be isolated in specialised laboratories by inoculation of laboratory animals or fertile eggs.

EPIDEMIC TYPHUS

Louse-borne or epidemic typhus caused by *Rickettsia prowazeki* is transmitted by infected faeces from the louse of man, usually through scratching the skin, but sometimes by inhalation. Patients suffering from epidemic typhus infect the lice, and these leave the patient if he is febrile. In conditions of overcrowding the disease may spread rapidly. During interepidemic periods the disease may be maintained by inapparent or latent cases ('Brill's disease') or perhaps by infected fleas and rats.

Pathology. Vascular changes in typhus are especially characteristic in the vessels of the brain. There may be increased pressure of the cerebrospinal fluid with excess of protein and lymphocytes. The white cell count is usually normal.

Clinical Features. The incubation period is usually 12 to 14 days. There may be a few days of malaise but the onset is more often sudden with rigors, frontal headaches and pains in the back and limbs. The temperature rises for two or three days, constipation is constant, and bronchitis usually distressing. The face is flushed and cyanotic, eyes congested, and the patient soon becomes dull and confused.

The rash appears on the fourth to the sixth day and often resembles measles. In its early stages it disappears on pressure but soon becomes petechial with subcutaneous mottling. It appears first on the anterior folds of the axillae, sides of the abdomen or back of hands, thence on the trunk and forearms. The neck and face are seldom affected.

During the second week symptoms increase in severity. Sordes collect on the lips, and the tongue, dry and brown, becomes shrunken and tremulous. The spleen becomes palpable, the pulse feeble and the patient stuporous and delirious. If the patient recovers, the temperature falls rapidly at the end of the second week and convalescence ensues. In fatal cases the patient usually dies in the second week from general toxaemia, heart or renal failure or pneumonia.

Common complications are bronchopneumonia, parotitis, venous thrombosis and gangrene.

Diagnosis. The clinical features may be almost diagnostic especially when there is an epidemic of the disease. In mild cases of the disease, however, clinical symptoms and signs may be much less distinctive. In the Weil-Felix test agglutination of Proteus OX 19 over 1/200 is usual after the seventh day; a rising titre is of particular diagnostic value. The complement-fixation test with a killed suspension of *R. prowazeki* gives reliable results and differentiates it from flea-borne typhus.

Measles, meningococcal septicaemia, malaria, relapsing fever, typhoid fever, smallpox and other fevers of the typhus group have to be differentiated.

Louse-borne typhus is notifiable under the International Sanitary Regulations.

ENDEMIC TYPHUS

Flea-borne or 'endemic' typhus is caused by *R. mooseri*, which on intraperitoneal inoculation of a guinea-pig, causes a febrile illness with a marked, often haemorrhagic, scrotal reaction (Neill-Mooser reaction).

This reaction is unusual in *R. prowazeki* infection. Man is infected when, by scratching, he introduces the faeces or contents of a crushed flea (*Xenopsylla astia* or *X. cheopis*) which has fed on an infected rat. The incidence of the disease is sporadic.

Pathology. Deaths are rare in human infections, so morbid changes, probably slighter than in louse-borne typhus, have not been studied in detail.

Clinical Features. The incubation period is 8 to 14 days. The symptoms resemble those of a mild louse-borne typhus. The rash may be scanty and transient.

Diagnosis. The Weil-Felix OX 19 is positive as in louse-borne typhus and the specific complement-fixation test using *R. mooseri* antigen is positive by the ninth day.

TICK-BORNE TYPHUS FEVERS
Rocky Mountain Spotted Fever

The causal organism, *R. rickettsi*, transferred by the bite of ticks, carries disease to rodents and dogs and on occasion to man when brought into contact with these animals. It is widely distributed in western and south-eastern States of the USA and also in South America.

Pathology. The vascular changes are similar to those in epidemic typhus. In addition, haemorrhages and gangrene of the genitalia, ears and digits sometimes occur and there may be bronchopneumonia and enlargement of the spleen and liver.

Clinical Features. The incubation period is about seven days. There may be an eschar at the site of the bite, with enlargement of the regional lymph nodes. Symptoms, which include severe headache, generalised pains and high fever falling by lysis during the third week, closely resemble those of louse-borne typhus. The rash appears about the third or fourth day, at first like measles, but in a few hours the typical maculo-papular eruption appears. Lesions, rose-red at first, become fainter with the morning remission of fever in the early stages. Each day, however, they become more distinct and papular until they are petechial. The rash first appears on the wrists, forearms and ankles, spreads in 24 to 48 hours to the back, limbs and chest and lastly to the abdomen where it is least pronounced. The fully developed rash often affects also the palms, soles and face. Petechiae may appear in crops. Cutaneous and subcutaneous haemorrhages of considerable size may appear in severe cases. Complications are as in louse-borne typhus. Untreated, the course of the disease may be mild or rapidly fatal.

Diagnosis. There may be a history of a bite by a tick. The character of the rash, appearing first at the periphery, is helpful. The rickettsiae can be isolated from the blood (p. 60). The Weil-Felix reaction is not of much help. Agglutination and complement-fixation tests using *R. rickettsi* antigen are positive in the second week.

Other Forms of Tick-borne Typhus

The causal agents of African tick-borne typhus are *R. conori* and a substrain, *R. conori pijperi*. They cause typhus in South and East Africa, the reservoir hosts being dogs and rodents. Fièvre boutonneuse of the Mediterranean is similar, as is also the infection in Queensland where *R. australis* is the causal organism. There are antigenic differences between these various rickettsiae. An eschar and lymphadenitis are usual. The rash is maculo-papular and may cover the trunk and limbs and affects the palms and soles. There may be delirium and meningeal signs in severe infections but recovery is the rule except in the debilitated. There are no haemorrhages into the skin. Positive results are obtained in the Weil-Felix test in the majority of cases but may be only to a low titre.

The infection may be acquired by walking on grasslands but in endemic areas dogs may bring the infected ticks into the house.

SCRUB TYPHUS

Mite-borne or 'scrub' typhus is caused by *R. tsutsugamushi* transmitted by the bite of infective larval mites, such as *Leptotrombidium (Leptotrombidium) akamushi* and *L. (L.) deliense*.

Geographical Distribution. Far East, Assam, Burma, West Pakistan, Indonesia, S. Pacific Islands and Queensland.

Pathology. This is similar to that of louse-borne typhus, but lesions in the lungs are more prominent. A primary eschar and necrosis of the superficial part of the dermal epithelium are correlated with mononuclear infiltration, phlebitis and intimal changes at the site of the bite.

Clinical Features. The incubation period is about nine days. In most cases an eschar, starting as a small papule, becomes a small rounded or oval ulcer up to 10 mm. in diameter surrounded by a red indurated area. Multiple eschars are seen not infrequently. The associated lymph nodes are often enlarged.

The onset of symptoms is usually sudden with headache, often retro-orbital, fever, malaise, weakness and cough, occasionally with diarrhoea. The conjunctivae become injected. In severe case the general symptoms increase, with apathy and prostration. A rash often appears on about the fifth to the seventh day, at first reddish macules on the front and back of the chest and on the abdominal wall. In twenty-four hours it becomes a raised maculo-papular rash which soon appears on the face, neck, arms, palms, legs and soles. The rash usually fades by the fourteenth day. The temperature rises rapidly and continues as a remittent fever with sweating until it falls by lysis about the twelfth to the eighteenth day. The fever and rash are frequently associated with generalised enlargement of lymph nodes which are firm, elastic, discrete and painless.

Cough and headaches are troublesome and mental change may be striking. By the tenth day the patient is prostrate, lethargic and querulous, distressed by cough and often deaf. The pulse, slow at first, becomes rapid in severe cases, and peripheral circulatory failure frequently precedes death. There are often signs of pneumonitis, especially towards the bases of the lungs. The sputum may be frothy and streaked with blood. Radiological changes in the lungs, when present, are similar to those found in virus pneumonia. In patients progressing to recovery the temperature falls by lysis, but convalescence is often slow and tachycardia may persist for some weeks. Mild cases show less severe symptoms and recovery is quicker.

Diagnosis. In endemic areas diagnosis is often possible on the clinical findings of fever, severe headache and congested conjunctivae. An eschar, rash, enlarged lymph nodes and mental changes give further assistance.

Enteric fever, malaria, leptospirosis and other forms of typhus must be excluded.

Isolation of rickettsiae by intraperitoneal inoculation of blood into mice during the first week is diagnostic. The Weil-Felix reaction with Proteus OXK starts after the seventh day and reaches a maximum two weeks later. Complement-fixation and agglutination tests using *R. tsutsugamushi* antigen are positive after the second week.

Q (Query) FEVER

The causative organism of this disease, which occurs throughout the world, differs sufficiently from other rickettsiae to be placed in a separate genus and is known as *Coxiella burneti*. Ticks of several genera are vectors of *C. burneti*, and these convey the infection to many wild animals and to large domestic animals. These organisms are very resistant to drying and so lend themselves to dissemination by air. Man may become infected by inhaling or ingesting infected dust, rarely, if ever, by the bite of a tick.

Dried genital discharges, milk and urine from infected animals appear to be important sources of infection amongst meat handlers and agricultural workers. Infected straw and other packing material have also been incriminated. Infections have been acquired in laboratory and autopsy rooms.

Clinical Features. The incubation period is 7 to 14 days. The onset is sudden with fever, sweating and general malaise, cough, retro-orbital pain and anorexia. The temperature rises from 39° to 40·5° C. (102° to 105° F.) with daily remissions, to fall to normal after 4 to 15 days. The pulse is slow, prostration often marked, and a dry cough is often present about the fifth or sixth day with scanty sputum, occasionally bloodstained. Pains in the chest are frequent, but physical signs are minimal—perhaps a few fine crepitations and slight dullness on percussion. The spleen is sometimes palpable and occasionally a sparse rash is present. Radiographs show patchy homogeneous ground-glass areas of consolidation, single or multiple, usually towards the base of the lungs. These usually resolve in about ten days. Occasionally the lung fields show no radiological change. Hepatitis, encephalitis and endocarditis with features resembling bacterial endocarditis are rare complications.

With the fall of temperature convalescence is usually rapid and complete.

Diagnosis. The clinical symptoms resemble those of virus pneumonia or of septicaemia. The Weil-Felix test is negative but, with a specific antigen from *C. burneti*, antibodies can be demonstrated in the second week and are maximal in the fifth or sixth week. The organisms can be recovered from the blood (p. 60).

RICKETTSIALPOX

This disease is due to *R. akari*, transmitted from the domestic mouse by a mite. It appears to be restricted to New York and Philadelphia where mice are now adapted to live in communal rubbish chutes of apartment houses.

Pathology. The lesions in the skin show necrosis of the capillary walls with thrombosis, perivascular lymphocytic infiltration and small haemorrhages. No lesions of other tissues have been observed, and the leucopenia is moderate.

Clinical Features. The first lesion starts as a deep-seated papule which gradually enlarges to form a rounded or oval vesicle. This eventually shrinks to a black eschar which separates after one to two weeks. The regional lymph nodes are usually enlarged.

About a week after the appearance of the first lesion fever, sweating and backache begin quite suddenly and continue for about a week.

The typical rash appears within the first four days of the fever. The lesions are red maculo-papules later forming vesicles at their centres. They soon dry to form black crusts which are shed after a few days leaving no permanent scars. There is no special site for the lesions, but they avoid the palms and soles. The patient is never seriously ill.

Diagnosis. The rickettsiae can be isolated from the blood during the acute stage (p. 60). The complement-fixation test with *R. akari* is positive.

TRENCH FEVER

Trench fever is caused by *R. quintana* and is spread to man by louse faeces. It was prevalent in the First World War in the trenches when troops were verminous and again in the Second World War in Russia.

Pathology. The disease is not fatal so the pathology is not well documented. Changes in the skin include hyperaemia, oedema and perivascular cellular infiltration without any typical vascular lesion.

Clinical Features. The incubation period is 10 to 20 days. The onset is sudden with headache, severe pains in trunk and limbs and tenderness in the back and legs, especially in the shins. The temperature rises sharply and remains continuously raised for five to seven days. Occasionally the fever is intermittent. Febrile relapses are common, usually at intervals of five to six days. Three to four such bouts may be expected. Tachycardia may be a feature. A rash, usually macular but occasionally papular, distributed mainly on the trunk, may appear on the second day of the fever and last only one day. It is rose red early and later becomes a dull red. The spleen is usually palpable. In chronic relapsing cases fatigue is often marked and convalescence may be prolonged for several months.

Diagnosis. In the presence of an outbreak the clinical picture of pains, rash and febrile relapses should suggest the diagnosis of trench fever. In addition to other rickettsial diseases, enteric fever, malaria, relapsing fever and brucellosis must be excluded.

Treatment of the Rickettsial Diseases

Specific Treatment. The various fevers due to rickettsiae vary greatly in severity but all respond to broad-spectrum antibiotics. Chloramphenicol was the first to be used and was dramatically successful. The typhus group, however, respond very well to tetracycline and, as aplastic anaemia is an occasional complication from chloramphenicol, it is wiser to use tetracycline. It is used in the standard dose, for an adult, of 250 mg. four times daily, but on the first day double this dose may be given. In severe infections the dose is 500 mg. four times daily for the first three days. The fever usually settles within two or three days. As the action of tetracycline is mainly bacteriostatic, there is a tendency to relapse and it should, therefore, be continued for five to seven days after the patient is afebrile.

General Management. The patient suffering from louse-borne or flea-borne typhus is a danger to others unless he has been disinfested.

When the temperature is high, sponging gives great comfort; for hyperpyrexia, i.e. over 41° C. (106° F.) sponging with cold or iced water is required. If headache is intense and fails to respond to aspirin or codeine, lumbar puncture should be performed to relieve the increased intracranial pressure and to detect any concomitant bacterial meningitis. Delirium may need to be controlled by sedatives while awaiting the effects of specific chemotherapy.

In scrub typhus pneumonitis may be a serious feature, and oxygen may be needed.

Convalescence is usually protracted especially in older people.

Prophylaxis. In louse and flea-borne typhus and in trench fever steps should be taken to get rid of all lice and fleas and their faeces. An insecticide powder can be insufflated into the undergarments of those at risk without their undressing. To prevent flea-borne typhus food stores and granaries should be protected from rats. Rats and their fleas must be destroyed.

Attendants on patients with louse-borne typhus should wear protective clothing smeared with an insect repellent such as dimethylphthalate (DMP). The patient should be washed, and an insecticide powder applied all over, especially to the hairy parts. His clothing should be immersed in disinfectant before being sterilised.

To guard against tick-borne typhus dogs should be regularly disinfested of ticks with forceps and should not be allowed to sleep in bedrooms. Protection of the legs when walking through grasslands may reduce the risk of picking up infected ticks. The early removal of ticks and cleansing the site of the bite are also important.

Mite-borne typhus is acquired when man enters scrub country in endemic areas. Protection against the larval mite can be secured by wearing suitable clothing, the inside of which has been smeared once a week with a mite-repellant such as DMP. Mites can be destroyed by aerial spraying of infected areas with Aldrin or Dieldrin, repeated every three months.

Active Immunisation. Those likely to be at risk can be protected against louse-borne and flea-borne typhus by Cox's vaccine prepared from killed cultures of strains of *R. prowazeki* and *R. mooseri* cultured in eggs. Three doses each of 1 ml. should be given subcutaneously at intervals of 7 to 10 days and when the risk is grave booster doses of 1 ml. should be given at six-monthly intervals. Cox's vaccine against infection with *R. rickettsi*, similarly prepared and administered, gives good protection. To maintain the immunity the vaccinations should be repeated annually.

So far no protective vaccine is available against mite-borne typhus.

Diseases due to Helminths

SCHISTOSOMIASIS (BILHARZIASIS)

THERE are three species of flukes of the genus *Schistosoma* which cause disease in man, *S. haematobium*, *S. mansoni* and *S. japonicum*. *S. haematobium* was discovered by Theodor Bilharz in Cairo in 1861 and the disease is sometimes called bilharziasis and the genus, *Bilharzia*. Certain other species, *S. intercalatum*, *S. bovis* and *S. matthei* only rarely affect man. When the ovum is passed in the urine or faeces and gains access to fresh water, the ciliated miracidium inside it is liberated and, if a suitable freshwater snail (p. 76) is available, it soon penetrates this intermediate host. In the snail in the hot season it develops into large numbers of forked-tailed cercariae which are then liberated into the water where they may survive for one to three days. These cercariae can penetrate the skin if there is only a thin film of water next to it, or the mucous membrane of the mouth of their definitive host, man; after passing to the lung they migrate to the portal vein where they reach maturity. The male worm is up to 20 mm. in length and the more slender cylindrical female, usually enfolded longitudinally by the male, is rather longer. Within four to six weeks of infection they migrate to the venules draining the pelvic viscera where the females deposit their ova. Whereas the eggs of *S. haematobium* are laid chiefly in the walls of the bladder and rectum, the eggs of *S. mansoni* and *S. japonicum* are deposited mainly in the lower bowel.

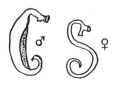

(Adults × 2½)

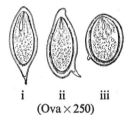

i   ii   iii
(Ova × 250)

FIG. 5

Schistosoma
i. *S. haematobium*
ii. *S. mansoni*
iii. *S. japonicum*

Pathology. Penetration of the skin by the cercariae may produce a papular eruption which may later become vesicular. A similar cutaneous eruption may, however, follow invasion of the skin by cercariae of schistosomes not otherwise pathogenic to man. During the migration of the immature schistosomes transitory lesions may be produced, including areas of pneumonitis. At this stage there is usually a considerable or great increase of eosinophils in the blood but the count falls progressively after the disease is established. In a heavy schistosomal infection ova may be found widely distributed in many tissues of the body, including the central nervous system, liver, lungs, heart and even the skin, but each species has a special territory for maximum egg deposition. After the egg has escaped from the vein, a granuloma forms around it. This consists of epithelioid cells, fibroblasts and giant cells surrounded by a zone of plasma cells and eosinophils. When the egg is near a mucosal surface, aided by the cytolytic enzyme excreted by the miracidium, it may be discharged into the bowel or bladder. If, however, the ovum is retained in the tissues the miracidium soon dies and the egg then either disintegrates or becomes calcified, and fibrous tissue forms at the site. The degree of fibrosis depends on the intensity of the infection and the length of time the patient has been exposed to re-infection. In endemic areas immune processes may limit re-infections.

Clinical Features. The first indication of infection, especially when it is heavy, may be tingling and itching of the part which has been exposed to water containing cercariae. This may last for one or two days and be succeeded, after a symptom-free period of three to five weeks, by allergic manifestations such as urticaria and eosinophilia and by fever, aches in the muscles, abdominal pain, splenomegaly, headaches, cough and sweating. Patches of pneumonic consolidation may be present. These allergic phenomena (Katayama syndrome) may be severe in infections with *S. mansoni* and *S. japonicum* but are rare with *S. haematobium*. After one or two weeks these features subside and for two or three months after the infection there may be no further symptoms until the deposition of eggs causes fresh ones to develop. The symptoms then depend on the intensity of the infection and the species of the infecting schistosome.

Schistosoma haematobium

This species of schistosome affects mainly the urinary bladder and the genitalia. The egg is easily recognised by its terminal spine. Man is the only natural host.

Geographical Distribution. *S. haematobium* is highly endemic in Egypt, the east coast of Africa and the adjacent islands and occurs throughout most of Africa, in Iran, Iraq, Syria, Yemen, South Arabia, Lebanon and Israel. It also occurs in Turkey, Cyprus and in solitary foci in Portugal and the Maharashtra State of India. *(NOT CARIBBEAN)*

Pathology. The urinary bladder and ureters are characteristically affected. The earliest changes in the mucosa are hyperaemia and petechiae, followed by small granulomata enlarging to form small papillomata but large granulomata may develop in young people. Sloughing may leave an ulcerated surface with associated fibrosis. Calcification of dead ova produces, in intense infections, 'sandy patches' especially towards the base of the bladder and around the ureteric openings. The lower third of the ureter, including its entrance into the bladder, is liable to stenosis causing partial obstruction to the passage of urine. In severe prolonged infections the bladder wall becomes extensively fibrosed and ultimately may calcify. The capacity of the bladder is greatly diminished. The increased intravesical pressure so produced leads to back-pressure on the kidneys and this alone or combined with ureteric obstruction produces hydro- or pyonephrosis and eventually extensive renal damage and uraemia. Calculus formation and pyogenic urinary infections may also ensue. Carcinoma of the bladder in relatively young males is of common occurrence in some areas of high endemicity of *S. haematobium*. Eggs may be deposited in the urethra, with sinus formation, in the seminal vesicles, vagina, cervix and Fallopian tubes, and this along with superadded pyogenic infection may lead to serious pelvic complications. The rectum may be involved, also the liver (periportal fibrosis), though less severely than in *S. mansoni* infections. Deposition of ova in the pulmonary arterioles may lead to hypertrophy of the inner and middle coats and cause partial or complete occlusion of some of these vessels. This will throw an additional strain on the right side of the heart and lead to cor pulmonale. These lung changes are especially frequent in combined infections with *S. haematobium* and *S. mansoni*. Ova may also be carried to the central nervous system, skin and elsewhere.

Clinical Features. The characteristic early localising symptom is usually terminal, painless haematuria with or without frequency of micturition. The haematuria is usually increased by exercise. When the disease has been established for some considerable time and the bladder has been damaged, all symptoms are increased with more haematuria and frequency due largely to the contracted fibrosed or calcified bladder. These symptoms, constant by day and night, may be very distressing. Pain at this stage is often felt in the iliac fossa or in the loin, passing down to the groin. In advanced cases pyelonephritis, hydro- or pyonephrosis may be accompanied by hypertension or may terminate in uraemia. Disease of the seminal vesicles may lead to haemospermia. In females fibrosis of the ovaries, occlusion of the Fallopian tubes and vaginitis or cervicitis may be produced, and schistosomal granulomata may be mistaken for carcinoma. Intestinal symptoms may result from lesions in the bowel wall.

The severity of *S. haematobium* infection varies greatly, and many with light infections suffer a minimum of discomfort. However, as the adult worms can live for 20 years or more and progressive lesions develop treatment should be given, even when infection is minimal.

Schistosoma mansoni

This species of schistosome affects characteristically the large bowel. The egg has a lateral spine. Man is the only natural host of importance although the infection is also found in baboons.

Geographical Distribution. *S. mansoni* is endemic in the Nile Delta and Libya, Southern Sudan, East Africa continuing as far south as the Transvaal and in West Africa from Senegal and Gambia to the Cameroons, throughout Congo and also in Arabia. It is also found in South America in Venezuela, Brazil and in the West Indian Islands of the lesser Antilles, Puerto Rico and Dominica.

Pathology. The adult worms reach the tributaries of the inferior mesenteric vein, and the female deposits eggs chiefly in the submucosa of the large bowel, producing early lesions similar to those caused in the bladder by *S. haematobium*—congested spots, granulomata and later papillomata. The papillomata in the bowel exceptionally become very large and pedunculated. They are most numerous in the lower part of the large bowel but may extend throughout its length. Occasionally a segment of the bowel wall becomes infiltrated and thickened but remains without stricture or malignant change. In long-standing severe infections rectal polypi may prolapse, and secondary pyogenic infection may create faecal fistulae. Eggs may be deposited throughout the body, in the mesenteric nodes, the small intestine and the subperitoneal tissues. In heavy infections the liver receives many eggs from the portal vein. This, in combination with toxic products from the adult schistosomes, may cause periportal fibrosis (pipe-stem cirrhosis) with granulomatous changes in the walls of the branches of the portal vein and subsequent periportal formation of vessels and connective tissue. In the early stage the liver is enlarged, firm, smooth and painless, but later it shrinks. The surface shows little or no irregularity. In advanced cases fibrosis leads to portal hypertension and ascites. The spleen is often slightly enlarged early in the disease, due to reticulo-endothelial proliferation, but with the development of hepatic fibrosis and portal hypertension the spleen may become very large and extremely hard. Pulmonary vascular lesions may be marked and lead to cor pulmonale. Eggs may reach the central nervous system and cause a granulomatous space-occupying lesion, the cord being the most usual site.

Clinical Features. The symptoms during the invasion by the cercariae and development of the adult worms have been described (p. 70). Depending on the intensity of the infection, symptoms due to deposition of eggs emerge after a period of two months or longer. The characteristic localising symptoms are abdominal pain and frequent stools which contain blood-stained mucus. The faecal matter is usually solid and its passage over the diseased mucosa causes trauma and bleeding. On palpation of the abdomen thickened infiltrated loops of the bowel may sometimes be detected. Where the mucosa of the lower bowel is severely affected, rectal polyps may prolapse during defaecation. Hepatosplenomegaly occurring early in the disease is reversible but in severe cases the liver becomes fibrotic and the spleen enlarged and hard, portal hypertension and ascites may develop and the patient dies of haematemesis, hepatic failure or secondary infection. Jaundice is not a frequent feature of this disease. Where infection is light no inconvenience may be experienced and the infection may be discovered only on routine examination of the stool. Other complications of *S. mansoni* infection include paraplegia from a lesion of the cord and, as described under pathology, cor pulmonale. In highly endemic areas the mortality from this disease is considerable.

Schistosoma japonicum

S. japonicum infects particularly the portal drainage of the small intestine and upper part of the large bowel. The egg has a lateral knob. The adult worm parasitises, in addition to man, the dog, rat, field mouse, water buffalo, ox, cat, pig, horse and sheep.

Geographical Distribution. *S. japonicum* is prevalent in the Yangtse-Kiang basin in China where the infection is a major public health problem. It also has a focal distribution in Japan and occurs in the Philippines, Celebes, Laos, Thailand, Vietnam and the Shan States of Burma.

Pathology. The histopathology of *S. japonicum* lesions is similar to that of the other schistosome diseases in man. As this worm produces more eggs the lesions tend to be more extensive and widespread. The small intestine and upper part of the large bowel are most affected, and hepatic fibrosis with splenic enlargement is usual. Deposition of eggs in the central nervous system, especially in the brain, causes symptoms of cerebral irritation or compression in about 5 per cent. of infections.

Clinical Features. The clinical features of schistosomiasis due to *S. japonicum* resemble those of very severe infection with *S. mansoni*. Dysenteric symptoms may be marked, and hepatic and splenic changes are usually early with ascites and the development of the superficial abdominal collateral venous circulation. Haematemesis and melaena may follow rupture of varicose veins in the stomach and oesophagus.

Neurological symptoms include Jacksonian epilepsy, hemiplegia, blindness and terminal coma. Evidence of compression of the cord may also be found.

The morbidity and mortality rate in *S. japonicum* infections is greater than from either of the other species.

Diagnosis of Schistosomiasis. A history of residence in an endemic area with symptoms as described will indicate the need for a careful investigation. An itch after contact with fresh water suggests the possible acquisition of this disease, especially if followed, after an interval, by allergic manifestations. In *S. haematobium* infection the terminal spined egg can usually be found by microscopical examination of the last few drops of urine, especially if brisk exercise has been undertaken by the patient before voiding the specimen. The eggs may also be found by microscopic examination of the stool or of a fragment of unstained rectal mucosa removed through a proctoscope. In a case of some duration a radiograph may show calcification of the wall of the bladder while intravenous pyelography may show stenosis or dilatation of the ureters, reduction in capacity of the bladder, or hydronephrosis. Such changes are found commonly in endemic areas and have been shown to be frequent even in children, in whom large intravesical granulomata are not uncommon. In a heavy infection with *S. mansoni* or *S. japonicum* the characteristic egg can usually be found in the stool. When, however, the infection is light it may be necessary to repeat the examinations over a number of days. Cystoscopy or sigmoidoscopy may enable the diagnosis to be made from the macroscopic appearance. Otherwise biopsy specimens should be removed and examined for ova. A complement-fixation reaction, using an alcoholic extract of fresh livers of *Planorbis boissyi* heavily infected with cercariae of *S. mansoni* as antigen, has proved of value in diagnosis, especially in the early stages of infection. The bowel symptoms of *S. mansoni* and *S. japonicum* infection may be very like those associated with intestinal amoebiasis or with a neoplasm of the large bowel, so steps should be taken to exclude these. There may be concomitant bacillary dysentery.

Treatment of Schistosomiasis. Sodium antimonyl tartrate is probably still the most reliable drug for all forms of schistosomiasis. · The intravenous route must be used, the greatest care being taken not to allow any of the solution to leak outside the vein, where it could cause intense tissue reaction and necrosis. Starting with 30 mg. the dose is doubled each day, if there are no ill-effects, up to a maximum of 120 mg. Each dose is diluted in 5 to 10 ml. of sterile water and the injection is given very slowly as this reduces the chances of toxic effects, such as cough, vomiting and even acute circulatory failure. If the side-effects are severe it may be advisable to give the dose on alternate days, diminish the daily dose or even discontinue this treatment. The total dosage to cure *S. mansoni* and *S. japonicum* infection is a minimum of 2 g., but for *S. haematobium* slightly less may be needed. The drug is given by 18 or more separate injections. The patient must rest in bed during the injection and for some hours afterwards. This is the only really satisfactory course of treatment for the cure of infection with *S. mansoni* and *S. japonicum*.

S. haematobium infections are more easily cured, and various preparations give reasonably satisfactory results. The efficacy of treatment may be assessed by the rate of reduction in the number of ova passed, as well as by their abolition.

An alternative form of trivalent antimony incorporating dimercaprol is stibocaptate. This is administered intramuscularly or by slow intravenous injection. The total dose, calculated as 40 to 50 mg./kg. body weight, is given in four or five divided doses during a period of four to eight days according to tolerance. Side-effects, vomiting, general depression and fever may be severe, especially if the solution has not been made up fresh for each injection.

Niridazole is administered by mouth in a dose of 25 mg./kg. body weight for seven days. Results, especially for *S. haematobium*, are reasonably good. Occasionally it produces a temporary psychosis. It is contra-indicated if the liver is diseased. The ease of its oral administration and the relatively satisfactory results obtained for *S. haematobium* infections have led to its widespread use.

Hycanthone (Etrenol), a new thioxanthone compound, is claimed to produce cure of a high percentage of *S. haematobium* and *S. mansoni* infections by a single intramuscular injection of 3 mg./kg. body weight (maximum dose 200 mg. of base).

Surgical aid may be required to deal with residual lesions but large vesical granulomata usually respond well to chemotherapy. In cases of chronic *S. haematobium* infection, ureteric stricture and the small fibrotic urinary bladder may require plastic procedures. For rectal papillomata removal by diathermy or by other means may give the patient considerable comfort. Granulomatous masses in the brain or spinal cord may call for neuro-surgery if the manifestations do not yield to chemotherapy. For portal hypertension splenectomy or a portocaval shunt operation may be necessary.

Preventive measures present great difficulties, and so far no really satisfactory means of controlling schistosomiasis has been discovered. If the ova of the schistosome in the urine or faeces are not allowed to contaminate fresh water containing the required snail host, then the miracidia will soon cease to be infective.

In a primitive country bore-hole latrines can easily be constructed but the great difficulty is to persuade the people always to use them. In the case of *S. japonicum*, moreover, there are so many hosts besides man that the proper use of latrines would be of little avail. Mass treatment of the population helps against *S. haematobium* and *S. mansoni* but this method has so far had little success against *S. japonicum*.

Attack on the intermediate host, the snail, presents many difficulties. The most important snail hosts of *S. haematobium* are species of the genus *Bulinus* and *Planorbarius*. In the case of *S. mansoni*, species of the genus *Biomphalaria*, *Australorbis* and *Tropicorbis* are the chief intermediate hosts. If an attempt is made to kill these snails by draining away the water in which they live they may preserve themselves by burrowing into the mud. In the Far East snails of the genus *Oncomelania* are the important intermediate hosts. They are very resistant to drying. Many molluscicides have been introduced into streams and canals in an attempt to destroy these snail hosts but so far without much success.

Personal Protection. Contact with infected water must be avoided. Accidental immersion or contact should be followed by a shower and one dose of intravenous sodium antimonyl tartrate. Water free from snails, stored for three days, will usually contain no living cercariae, but exceptions to this rule have been reported.

CLONORCHIASIS

Clonorchiasis results from infection of the bile ducts by the trematode *Clonorchis sinensis*. This is a flat elongated worm about 4 cm. long which produces numerous ova 19×16 microns in size. Dogs, cats and pigs may be infected in addition to man. The eggs are passed in the faeces. To complete the life cycle the eggs must be ingested by a freshwater snail and then the cercariae which escape from it enter a freshwater fish. If this fish is eaten raw or insufficiently cooked, man becomes infected.

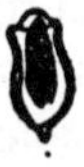

FIG. 6
Clonorchis sinensis
Ovum × 250.

Geographical Distribution. The infection occurs in China, Korea, Taiwan, Japan and Vietnam but is more prevalent in South China.

Pathology. Light infections do little harm. With heavier infections there is a proliferation of biliary epithelium and stagnation of bile predisposing to recurrent cholangitis due to *Escherichia coli*. Pseudocysts containing the worms may form in the bile ducts. The complications are abscesses in the liver arising from cholangitis, carcinoma of the biliary duct, and cirrhosis of the liver. Cholangitis, associated with the death of numerous worms may present as an attack of hypoglycaemia. Occasionally the pancreatic duct is dilated and contains many worms, the presence of which predisposes to attacks of acute pancreatitis.

Clinical Features. In the endemic areas ova are often found in the stools without symptoms being present. In other cases the presence of the worms is associated with epigastric pain of gradual onset or recurrent attacks of fever, pain and jaundice from complicating cholangitis or the symptoms and signs of the complications detailed above.

Diagnosis. The finding of ova in the stool or fluid aspirated from the duodenum establishes the presence of the worms but not necessarily the cause of the epigastric pain or other symptoms. Ova are sometimes scanty and only intermittently excreted.

Treatment. Treatment in the past has been unsatisfactory but hexachloroparaxylol (Chloxyle) 250 mg./kg. body weight twice daily on alternate days for 20 doses is now claimed to be effective. When secondary suppurative cholangitis ensues, an appropriate antibiotic should be given and surgical drainage may be required.

Prevention. Fish should be properly cooked before being eaten by man or fed to dogs, cats or pigs.

PARAGONIMIASIS
(Endemic Haemoptysis)

This disease is caused by a small trematode. There are several species of *Paragonimus* which may affect man, the commonest being *P. westermani*. The adult worms live in small cysts in the lung and elsewhere. If a pulmonary cyst ruptures, the sputum of the patient contains ova, some of which may be expectorated and the others swallowed and passed in the faeces. From these eggs the larval worms emerge in water and seek the first intermediate host, a freshwater snail. Larvae emerging from the snail enter freshwater crabs or crayfish. If man or certain other mammals eat these crustacea raw or inadequately cooked, infection takes place.

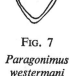

FIG. 7

Paragonimus westermani Ovum × 250.

Geographical Distribution. Human infections are most frequent in the Far East but there are also endemic foci in South America, Cameroons, Somalia and India.

Pathology. The adults lie in cysts up to 1 cm. in diameter, containing reddish brown fluid, situated chiefly in the lung. There are seldom more than 20 such cysts present. In heavy infections cysts may also be present in the pleural or peritoneal cavities, in the brain, muscles, skin or elsewhere.

Clinical Features.   The first symptoms are usually those of slight fever, cough and the expectoration of sputum streaked with blood.   Occasionally there are bouts of frank haemoptysis with severe pain in the chest.   Increasing signs in the chest may simulate pneumonitis or pulmonary tuberculosis and the latter frequently is a co-existent infection.   When the parasites lodge in the abdomen there may be symptoms of enteritis or hepatitis. If they settle in the abdominal wall they may produce sinuses with a discharge through the skin.   Development in the central nervous system may cause signs of cerebral irritation, encephalitis or myelitis.   The disease may be very chronic and the adult worms may survive for 20 years.

Diagnosis.   Ova may be found on microscopic examination of the faeces, sputum, or a discharge.   The radiological appearances of affected lungs are variable but the lesions are usually situated close to the pleural surfaces.   Extrapulmonary lesions are diagnosed in life by biopsy.

Treatment.   Antibiotics are useful to combat secondary pyogenic infections.   The specific drug is bithionol (2,2' thiobis (4,6 dichlorophenol)) given in a dose of 50 mg./kg. body weight daily in three divided doses on alternate days.   In all, 10 to 15 days of treatment are required and the results are encouraging.   Hexachloroparaxylol is also claimed to be effective (p. 77).   Lesions localised to or maximal in one lobe of a lung may be treated surgically.

Prevention.   In an endemic area crab or crayfish should not be eaten unless adequately cooked.   Immersion of infected crustaceans in wine or brine does not kill the parasites.

FASCIOLIASIS

Fasciola hepatica, the liver fluke of sheep, occasionally infects man. It is of historic interest that its presence in sheep was described by Jehan de Brie in 1379.   The adult worms, which live in the bile ducts, resemble small leaves approximately 3 cm. in length. Ova are passed in the sheep's droppings.   In water the miracidium escapes from the ovum and enters a snail of the genus *Lymnaea*, from which cercariae emerge to encyst, as metacercariae, on watercress or other aquatic plants, the consumption of which leads to infection.   The metacercariae penetrate the intestinal wall, peritoneal cavity and liver to mature in the biliary passages.

Fig. 8

F. hepatica

(adult)

Geographical Distribution.   The infection in sheep is cosmopolitan. Human infections are relatively common in North Africa and occasionally occur in Britain, especially in Hampshire, after unusually wet summers.

Pathology. The penetration of the liver by immature worms is associated with toxaemia and causes inflammatory changes and areas of necrosis and fibrosis. Numerous adult worms in the bile ducts lead to cystic dilation of the ducts and the formation of adenomata. Secondary to these changes, and superadded cholangitis, portal fibrosis may ensue. Inflammatory reactions also occur around ectopic worms.

Clinical Features. Symptoms and signs may be only those of an obscure low-grade fever associated with a tender enlarged liver and an eosinophilia. In heavier infections biliary colic, diarrhoea and signs of toxaemia may occur. Ectopic flukes may give rise to a nodule in the skin or signs of a lesion in the brain or elsewhere. 'Halzoun' (p. 109) was formerly attributed to *F. hepatica*.

Diagnosis. Ova may be found on examination of the faeces or duodenal aspirate but repeated examinations may be necessary. An eosinophilia is to be expected. A complement-fixation test is of some value but there is a cross reaction with *Fasciolopsis buski*.

Treatment. A course of chloroquine (150 mg. base) twice daily for 14 days may relieve the symptoms but injections of emetine hydrochloride, 60 mg. daily for six days, are more effective in overcoming the infection. Hexachloroparaxylol (p. 77) is claimed to be effective. Bithionol (p. 78) has recently been used successfully.

Prevention. In endemic areas, watercress should not be eaten.

FASCIOLOPSIASIS

Fasciolopsis buski is the largest trematode to infect man. It was first found in a sailor from the Far East by Busk in 1843 in London. It is ovoid, 2 to 7·5 cm. × 1 to 2 cm. and of a reddish colour. The adults inhabit the small intestine of man, of pigs and occasionally of dogs. Ova are passed in the faeces. In water the miracidia escape and invade a suitable snail, e.g. species of *Segmentina* from which cercariae emerge and give rise to metacercariae which encyst on edible water plants such as water caltrop or water chestnut. Infection is particularly liable to occur when man uses his teeth to peel the parasitised plants.

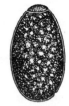

Fig. 9

F. buski

Ovum × 250

Geographical Distribution. The infection is common in Central and South China and amongst Chinese in South-East Asia.

Pathology. Localised inflammatory changes occur in the mucosa of the upper part of the small intestine. A moderate degree of eosinophilia is common.

Clinical Features. Light infections are usually symptomless. In heavier infections first there is epigastric pain resembling a peptic ulcer, later loose motions containing undigested food are passed. In very heavy infections, particularly in children, generalised oedema may develop and death ensue.

Diagnosis. Ova and occasionally adults are detected in the faeces. A complement-fixation test gives also a cross reaction with *Fasciola hepatica*.

Treatment. The usual treatment has been tetrachloroethylene as prescribed for hookworms but hexachloroparaxylol (p. 77) used as a single dose of 0·5 g./kg. body weight repeated once two weeks later has recently been employed successfully.

Prevention. The use of fresh human excreta on the fields is responsible for much of the spread of this infection. Prolonged storage of faeces or their treatment with quicklime, destroys the ova or immature worms. Edible water plants may be freed of metacercariae by immersing them in boiling water.

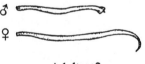

Adults × 2

Ovum × 250

Fig. 10

Ancylostoma duodenale

ANCYLOSTOMIASIS
(Hookworm Infection)

Ancylostomiasis is caused by parasitisation of the small intestine with *Ancylostoma duodenale* or *Necator americanus*. The adult hookworm is a greyish-white nematode about 1 cm. in length, approximately the size of a threadworm. The egg is thin-shelled and oval, slightly smaller than that of *Ascaris lumbricoides* and when passed in the faeces two to eight lobes may be seen in the yolk. In warm moist soil the larvae develop and reach the filariform infective stage. On coming in contact with human skin they penetrate it and are carried to the lungs. After entering the alveoli they ascend the bronchi, are swallowed and develop in the small intestine, reaching maturity in four to seven weeks after infection. The larvae may also enter through the mucous membrane of the mouth. Man is the only host.

Geographical Distribution. Hookworm infection is widespread under insanitary conditions in the tropics and subtropics and occurs in certain mines in Europe. *A. duodenale* is endemic in the Far East and Mediterranean coastal regions and is also present elsewhere in Africa. *N. americanus* is endemic in West, East and Central Africa and Central and South America as well as in the Far East.

Pathology. At the site of entry the larvae may cause a minor inflammatory and allergic reaction while bacterial infection may raise pustules. When infection is heavy, reaction to the passage through the lungs may cause a patchy inflammation with areas of pulmonary consolidation accompanied by eosinophilia. In the small intestine the worms attach themselves to the mucosa by their buccal capsule and withdraw blood. The mean daily loss of blood from one *A. duodenale* is 0·15 ml. but for *N. americanus* only 0·03 ml. The degree of iron deficiency which develops depends not only on the load of worms but also on the nutrition of the patient and especially on his stores of iron. In those on an adequate diet regeneration of red blood cells may keep pace with blood loss so that no anaemia may result (p. 141). In the early stage of infection a considerable eosinophilia commonly occurs.

Clinical Features. In a well nourished person there may be no symptoms, the infection being discovered only during a routine examination of the stool. At the time of infection hookworm dermatitis (ground itch) may be experienced, usually on the feet but it may be on any part of the body which has been in contact with infected soil. An itchy erythema appears first and soon develops through papules and vesicles to the pustular stage. In a heavy infection the passage of the larvae through the lungs may cause a cough with blood-stained sputum, associated with patchy pulmonary consolidation (an example of Loeffler's syndrome). When the worms have reached the small intestine, vomiting and epigastric pain, like that of a duodenal ulcer, may ensue. Sometimes frequent loose stools are passed, the condition then resembling early sprue or giardiasis. In the undernourished, especially when there is a heavy infection, a severe iron deficiency anaemia may develop. This is particularly the case in children in whom the appearance may simulate the nephrotic syndrome and kwashiorkor, there being often a puffy face, oedema of the extremities and a distended abdomen, sometimes with ascites. Tachycardia and breathlessness are present in those with severe anaemia. In children mental and physical development may be retarded. Infection with *A. duodenale* usually causes severe symptoms more readily than does infection with *N. americanus*. Concomitant malaria or other infections aggravate the ill effects of ancylostomiasis. Untreated heavy infections in the poorly nourished are responsible for many deaths.

Diagnosis. Iron deficiency anaemia in someone who has been exposed to the risk of hookworm infection demands a stool examination to exclude this disease. The characteristic egg can be recognised in the stool either by microscopic examination of a smear of the faeces directly or after concentration. Pulmonary symptoms similar to those present in the invasive phase of ancylostomiasis may also be produced by the larvae of *Ascaris lumbricoides, Schistosoma* or *Strongyloides* passing through the lungs. The oedema with anaemia has to be differentiated from that due to kwashiorkor, heart failure or nephritis. Hookworms may be present without being the chief agents responsible for symptoms and signs produced by concomitant associated disease. If hookworms are present in numbers sufficient to cause anaemia, tests of the stool for occult blood will be positive and ova will be present in large numbers.

Treatment. SPECIFIC. The vermicidal effect of most drugs is greatest when the upper bowel is empty. Accordingly treatment should be given early in the morning when the patient has fasted overnight. A well established drug is tetrachloroethylene which is given orally. The dose is 0·1 ml./kg. body weight with a maximum of 4 ml. The drug has usually to be given on two or more occasions not more frequently than on alternate days. Tetrachloroethylene rapidly deteriorates in warm climates and so must be stored in a cool dark place.

Bephenium hydroxynaphthoate, a quaternary ammonium compound, is an alternative drug with few side effects. The dose, irrespective of age, is 5 g., containing 2·5 g. base, as a single dose. No preparation or purgation is required. A further dose is necessary for those who continue to pass ova. It is more expensive than tetrachloroethylene and is not as effective for *N. americanus* as for *A. duodenale*.

NON-SPECIFIC. The irritation of ground itch can be relieved by the application of an ointment containing zinc oxide and salicylic acid. Anaemia associated with hookworm infection responds well to treatment with iron in adequate doses (p. **840**). A well balanced diet containing meat and vegetables is desirable. Where the anaemia is very severe, it should be corrected with iron or blood transfusion before giving an anthelmintic. In the presence of marked oedema transfusion is not free from the danger of causing left ventricular failure. Hence packed cells rather than whole blood should be employed and the transfusion given very slowly. Preliminary digitalisation may be desirable.

Prevention. Education of the population in the use of latrines should be arranged. Bore-hole latrines can be provided in suitable locations near villages. These should have concrete plinths so as to avoid contamination of the soil in the immediate vicinity of the latrine. When the infection is heavy, mass treatment of the entire population by tetrachloroethylene or bephenium hydroxynaphthoate is indicated, repeated periodically until the disease has been brought under control. The nutrition of the population should be improved. Where practicable the use of shoes should be encouraged.

STRONGYLOIDIASIS

Strongyloides stercoralis is a very small nematode (2 mm. $\times$ 40 microns) which parasitises the mucosa of the upper part of the small intestine in large numbers. The eggs hatch in the bowel and appear in the faeces as rhabditiform larvae which in moist soil moult and become the infective filariform larvae. These, on entering the tissues of man, undergo a development cycle similar to that of ancylostome larvae. Larvae sometimes mature in the lung. In the intestine a few rhabditiform larvae develop into filariform larvae which may then penetrate the mucosa or the perianal skin and lead to auto-infection. Man is the chief natural host, but dogs and cats may also be infected naturally.

Geographical Distribution. It is world-wide in the tropics and subtropics and is especially prevalent in the Far East.

Pathology. There may be a dermatitis at the time of entry of the larval worm, similar to that which may accompany invasion by ancylostome larvae. In the intestine the female worm burrows into the mucosa and sets up an inflammatory reaction; with very heavy infections the mucosa may be severely damaged leading to malabsorption. Granulomatous changes, necrosis, and even perforation and peritonitis may also occur. An increase in the total white cell count with a marked eosinophilia is common in the early stages and this may persist. Actively motile larvae are found in the faeces and occasionally in the sputum.

Clinical Features. An itch may be produced during invasion of the skin. Pulmonary symptoms and signs similar to those of ancylostomiasis may also occur. With slight infections there will be no intestinal symptoms, but in more severe cases abdominal pain and diarrhoea may be produced, which is on occasions severe; urticaria, anaemia, weakness and emaciation may also be present as well as signs of malabsorption, ileus or volvulus. Penetration of the skin about the anus or the intestinal wall by filariform larvae may lead to extremely itchy, linear, urticarial skin reactions. These usually subside in a few hours but tend to keep on recurring. The eruptions may extend 3 or 4 cm. in an hour. This rapid progress has led to the term 'larva currens' being used rather than 'larva migrans' or creeping eruption. In addition there are frequently urticarial wheals or less well defined areas of erythema. These eruptions appear to be rare in indigenous peoples. Filariform larvae may reach the brain and cause cerebral irritation.

Diagnosis. Intestinal symptoms and characteristic eruptions should suggest *S. stercoralis* infection. Eosinophilia is usually present. Under the low power of the microscope motile rhabditiform larvae can be seen in the faeces, occasionally in the sputum, urine or bile. Excretion of them is intermittent so repeated examinations may be necessary. In ancylostomiasis ova, not larvae, are found in a fresh stool. The larva migrans of the dog or cat ancylostome (see below) is located in the superficial layers of the skin and appreciable advancement of the serpiginous dermal lesion takes days, not minutes, as is the case with infection with strongyloides.

Treatment. Thiabendazole (2-(4'-Thiazolyl)-benzimidazole) given orally in a dose of 25 mg./kg. body weight twice daily for two to four days, according to its tolerance, produces a high percentage of cures. Some recurrent urticaria may continue for a time and a second similar course of thiabendazole may be required.

LARVA MIGRANS

Symptoms may result from various larval nematodes penetrating the tissues of man in whom development to mature worms cannot take place. Dermal lesions may be caused by the larvae of *Ancylostoma braziliense* or *A. caninum* of the cat or dog invading human skin, especially the skin of children. The larva burrows between the corium and stratum granulosum and progresses very slowly and irregularly, the advancing end showing a skin reaction with redness while the older part of the burrow is pale and scaly. These larvae may remain alive and active for several weeks. Treatment by freezing the advancing end with ethyl chloride or carbon dioxide snow is not always successful unless frequently repeated. Thiabendazole in a dose of 50 mg./kg. body weight for three doses at intervals of 12 hours or as already described above may succeed.

Infection with *Strongyloides stercoralis* may be associated with an eruption attributed to its larvae which travels so quickly (p. 83) that the name 'larva currens' is appropriate for it.

In the Far East (India, Thailand and China) human infection with the third stage larva of *Gnathostoma spinigerum*, which normally infects dogs and cats, may follow ingestion of raw fish or water containing infected *Cyclops*. Then the immature worm, measuring 6 mm. × 0·8 mm. usually migrates to the subcutaneous tissue where it causes recurrent swellings. The geographical distribution of this infection distinguishes it from loiasis in which similar 'Calabar' swellings are a feature. The full grown adult worm, which may be as long as 3 cm., may develop in man. When the worm, usually single, is visible through the skin it can be removed surgically. During migration in the deeper tissues the worm may cause injury to the brain, kidney, lung, eye or other organs. Eosinophilia is usually pronounced. Diagnosis is easy when the adult worm is visible. Otherwise complement-fixation tests, using a specific antigen, if available, will be required. Treatment is not fully satisfactory but some success has been obtained with bithional (p. 78).

The eggs of *Toxocara canis*, the common roundworm of dogs, may be passed in the faeces and be swallowed by children, causing visceral larva migrans. Puppies are infected prenatally through the placenta, the larvae migrating through the lung to the upper part of the intestinal tract. There they mature and produce enormous numbers of ova which are excreted in the faeces for about six months when the adult worms die. If young children ingest the eggs, somatic migration occurs and the larvae may remain alive in the tissues for years, causing minute granulomatous lesions. This visceral infection in children may produce the syndrome of fever, pulmonary infiltration, hepatomegaly, eosinophilia, hypergamma-globulinaemia and occasionally encephalopathy. The larvae sometimes reach the eye via the retinal circulation and cause a retinal granuloma about the disc or macula, or they may enter the vitreous body. Blindness of the affected eye may result. There is serological evidence that *T. canis* infection may predispose to epilepsy and paralytic poliomyelitis. A skin test, using an antigen from *T. canis*, is available for diagnosis. Rarely adult worms develop in the intestine.

Toxocara cati is regarded as another possible cause of visceral larva migrans in man.

Diethylcarbamazine (p. 89) may give satisfactory results in the treatment of larva migrans due to *Toxocara*, but preventive measures are all-important. Dogs, especially puppies, should be treated, to remove intestinal worms, and puppies should not be allowed to defaecate where children are likely to play.

Eosinophilic lung, as it occurs in the tropics (tropical pulmonary eosinophilia) is now commonly attributed to an abnormal host reaction to filarial larvae (p. 95).

FILARIASIS

INTRODUCTION

A number of different nematodes of the family *Filariidae* affect man. The adults are thin worms varying from 2 to 50 cm. in length and the larvae or microfilariae are easily visible under the low power of the microscope, being about 250 microns long. The mature females are viviparous. The adults of the species *Wuchereria bancrofti* and *Brugia malayi* inhabit and tend to block lymphatic vessels. Adult filariae of the species *Loa loa* wander in the subcutaneous tissue and cause Calabar swellings. The adults of *Onchocerca volvulus* may be surrounded by fibrous tissue in subcutaneous nodules but it is their larvae which cause a dermatosis and sometimes serious lesions in the eye. The larvae of *Dipetalonema streptocerca* may produce a similar but milder dermatosis but *Dipetalonema perstans* and *Mansonella ozzardi*, the larvae of which circulate in the blood, are non-pathogenic. The microfilariae have distinguishing morphological appearances (p. 87). It should be noted that the microfilariae of *Wuchereria*, *Brugia* and *Loa* are sheathed, the remainder unsheathed.

Wuchereria filariasis

Wuchereria bancrofti is conveyed to man by the bites of infected mosquitoes of a number of different species, the most common being *Culex fatigans*. The adult worms, 4 to 10 cm. in length, live in the lymphatics of man, and the females produce microfilariae which at night circulate in large numbers in the peripheral blood. As *Culex fatigans* bites at night the nocturnal periodicity of the microfilariae, first demonstrated by Manson in 1877, facilitates the spread of the infection. In some of the Pacific islands there is a non-periodic strain of *W. bancrofti* maintained by mosquitoes which bite in the day-time. When not circulating in the peripheral blood, the microfilariae are chiefly in the capillaries in the lungs.

Geographical Distribution. The infection is widespread in tropical Africa, the North African coast, coastal areas of Asia, Indonesia and Northern Australia, South Pacific Islands, West Indies and also in North and South America.

Pathology. The microfilariae do not harm the human host. Light infections may remain symptomless but are likely to be associated with an eosinophilia. In more intense and repeated infections the presence of mature worms in the lymphatic vessels and nodes leads to granulomatous changes and allergic tissue responses with infiltration of eosinophils around the lymphatics. These cellular changes are associated with attacks of lymphangitis and lead to temporary lymphatic obstruction. Eventually, after repeated attacks, in some of which secondary bacterial infections may play a part, permanent obstruction of a main lymphatic trunk may be produced. Progressive enlargement of the limb or region below the obstruction then follows with thickening and fibrosis of the tissues.

Clinical Features. After an incubation period of not less than three months the first manifestations are bouts of fever accompanied by pain

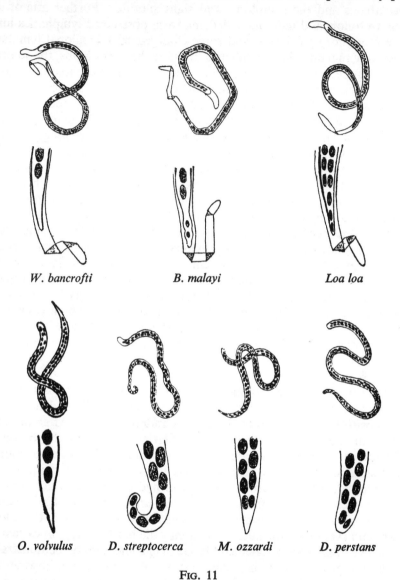

W. bancrofti   B. malayi   Loa loa

O. volvulus   D. streptocerca   M. ozzardi   D. perstans

FIG. 11

Microfilariae (×250)

Second and fourth rows show tails (greatly enlarged)

and tenderness along the course of inflamed lymphatic vessels over which there is cutaneous erythema. In addition there may be some scattered

D

urticaria. Inflammation of the spermatic cord (funiculitis), epididymitis and orchitis may be caused by lymphangitis. After a few days the fever abates and the symptoms and signs subside. Further attacks are likely to follow and temporary oedema from obstructed lymphatics tends to become more persistent, and some enlargement of regional lymphatic nodes may remain. The lymphatics draining the lower limbs, the scrotum and the upper limbs are those most frequently affected, mainly or only in one site in any one individual. The earlier effects may be the formation of superficial lymph varices, enlargement of lymph nodes and the production of hydroceles. Permanent obstruction of the main lymphatic trunks of a limb causes progressive enlargement, coarsening, corrugation and fissuring of the skin and subcutaneous tissue, with warty superficial excrescences, until a leg resembles that of an elephant. The name 'elephantiasis' is thus applied to this condition which may also occur in an upper limb, the scrotum, vulva or breast. The scrotum may reach an enormous size, a weight of 20 kg. or more being attained in some who remain ambulant. Obstruction of the abdominal lymphatics may lead to chyluria or chylous ascites. The interval between infection and the onset of elephantiasis is usually not less than 10 years, after which the condition tends to be slowly but remorselessly progressive, although minor degrees may persist unchanged. Gross elephantiasis only develops commonly in inhabitants of highly endemic areas where there is no control of mosquitoes. Those who are not well endowed with collateral lymphatics are especially prone to develop elephantiasis.

Diagnosis. In the earliest stages of lymphangitis the diagnosis is made on clinical grounds, supported usually by an eosinophilia and sometimes by a positive complement-fixation or intradermal test. After about a year from the time of infection microfilariae appear in the blood at night and can be seen moving in a wet blood film and identified in stained blood smears. They may also be found in the absence of symptoms in some people. They are usually present in hydrocele fluid which may on occasion yield an adult filaria. With the establishment of permanent elephantiasis it becomes unusual for microfilariae to reach the blood stream and eventually the adult worms may die but the lymphatics remain obstructed. Shadows of calcified filariae may sometimes be demonstrable by radiography. An initial exaggeration of symptoms following the administration of the specific drug, diethylcarbamazine, is indicative of a filarial infection.

COMPLEMENT-FIXATION TEST. This is a group reaction given by all pathogenic filariae. The antigen is usually prepared from *Dirofilaria immitis* or *Setaria cervi*, filariae of animal origin. This test is only positive in a proportion of cases but is rather more reliable, when positive, than an intradermal test using antigens of the same origin.

Treatment. Diethylcarbamazine, given orally, has a rapid destructive effect on microfilariae and a slower action against adult filariae. The dosage is up to 9 to 12 mg./kg. body weight daily in three divided doses for 21 days. The full dosage should, however, only be reached slowly, starting with 50 mg. (one tablet) and doubling daily if no untoward allergic responses ensue. This course may be repeated twice at intervals of four to six weeks. To control allergic phenomena antihistamines or, if necessary, corticosteroids may be required. Treatment with diethylcarbamazine, given early in the disease, produces cure and may lead to some amelioration in the more recently established cases of elephantiasis. In long-standing elephantiasis a prolonged course of corticosteroids is occasionally beneficial. Failing this, plastic surgery, preferably after preliminary radiological investigation of the lymphatics, is indicated. Great relief may be obtained by removal of excess tissue but recurrences are probable unless new lymphatic drainage is established. Tight bandaging, or bed rest with suspension or raising of the affected part, by reducing the swelling, will give temporary relief and may be desirable as a pre-operative measure.

Prevention. In endemic areas treatment of the whole population with diethylcarbamazine, 100 mg. for adults (50 mg. for children) three times daily for seven days, has reduced infection by robbing the mosquitoes of fresh sources of microfilariae. Children are given such a course on starting and just before leaving school. This mass treatment should be combined with control of the vector by insecticides (p. 1113). Personal protection is obtained by the wearing of protective clothing and the use of insect repellents. Where the vector is a night-biting mosquito wire-screening of the house or the use of mosquito nets prevents infection. Early chemotherapy prevents later elephantiasis.

Brugia filariasis

Brugia malayi resembles *W. bancrofti* closely. The microfilaria has distinguishing features and its sheath stains pink more readily with Giemsa's stain than the sheath of *W. bancrofti*. The microfilariae usually exhibit nocturnal periodicity but a semi-periodic form, which may affect man, commonly infects animals. A similar filaria, *Brugia pahangi*, is found chiefly in animals but has been transmitted to man. It, or a similar filaria, may be responsible for some cases of tropical eosinophilia (p. 95). The vectors of *B. malayi* are mosquitoes mostly belonging to the genus *Mansonioides*, the larvae of which draw air from the underwater stems of water hyacinths or mangroves.

Geographical Distribution. *B. malayi* is found in Indonesia, Borneo, Malaysia, Vietnam, South China, South India and Ceylon.

The pathology, clinical manifestations, treatment and personal prophylaxis are the same as those recorded for *W. bancrofti* except that elephantiasis is usually limited to the legs.

Prevention. A selective weed-killer, phenoxylene, has been used with success to rid ponds of the water hyacinth and thus to prevent *Mansonioides* from breeding.

Loiasis

Loiasis is caused by infection with the filaria *Loa loa*. The adults, 3 to 7 cm. long, parasitise chiefly the subcutaneous tissue of man. The larval microfilariae circulate harmlessly in the peripheral blood in the day-time, thus showing, in contrast to *W. bancrofti*, a diurnal periodicity. This led Manson in 1895 to postulate that the vector would be a fly biting by day, such as *Chrysops*, species of which are now known to convey the infection. A morphologically similar parasite infects monkeys but is not readily conveyed to man.

Geographical Distribution. Loiasis may be acquired in West Africa, Southern Sudan, Congo and Angola. It is endemic only in and around equatorial rain-forests.

Pathology. The adult worms move about in the subcutaneous tissues and other interstitial planes. Usually there is little evidence, apart from an eosinophilia, of a reaction of the hosts' tissues but from time to time a short-lived oedematous swelling (a Calabar swelling) is produced, presumably around an adult worm. Calcification of a dead worm is occasionally evident. Encephalitis has been attributed to microfilariae of *Loa loa* on rare occasions.

Clinical Features. The incubation period is commonly over a year but may be as short as three months. The infection may be symptomless. The first sign is often a Calabar swelling. This is felt as a somewhat irritating tense localised swelling which is painful only if it is near a joint. The swelling is generally on a limb; it measures a few centimetres in diameter but sometimes is more diffuse and extensive. It usually disappears after a few days but may persist for two or three weeks. Almost invariably a succession of such swellings appears at irregular intervals, often in near-by sites. Sometimes there is some urticaria and pruritus elsewhere. Occasionally a worm may be distinctly seen wriggling under the skin, especially of an eyelid and may cross the eye under the conjunctiva, taking many minutes to do so, sometimes causing irritation. When an adult worm is moving in retro-orbital tissues severe unilateral headache resembling migraine is experienced. Encephalitis due to *Loa loa* is probably a rare response to the death of numerous microfilariae particularly at the onset of treatment, especially if adult worms are situated in proximity to the eye.

Diagnosis. A reliable history of the crossing of the eye by a worm or of characteristic Calabar swellings in one who has resided in an endemic area enables a clinical diagnosis to be made. This will usually be supported by a considerable eosinophilia. The demonstration of microfilariae of *Loa loa* in the blood (or the recovery of an adult from the skin or eye) establishes the diagnosis. Some infections may be too recent for microfilariae to have reached the blood and in many they are scanty or intermittent in appearance. To demonstrate them a drop of blood, taken at midday, should be examined as a wet film under a coverslip. Microfilariae can be seen actively moving and it may be possible to detect the sheath. Examination of a stained blood film confirms the morphology. When microfilariae are scanty, concentration methods are useful. The filarial complement-fixation test (p. 88) is positive in 80 per cent. of infections and the intradermal test is usually positive. These are not specific for loiasis (p. 88).

Treatment. Diethylcarbamazine (p. 89) gradually increased to a dose of 9 to 12 mg./kg. body weight daily and continued at that dosage for 21 days is curative in most cases. Before diethylcarbamazine was available the removal of a worm crossing the eye or moving under the skin was practised but as other adult worms are almost invariably present this can no longer be recommended. Caution in treatment is particularly required if there is concomitant onchocerciasis (p. 92).

Prevention. For prevention a knowledge of the habits of the fly is important. The fly is attracted by a well-lit room, by movements of persons and also by wood smoke in native huts. Clearings in the forest of 100 to 200 yards act as a barrier to *C. silacea*. The most favoured breeding places are the mud flats covered with decaying vegetation bordering slow-running streams. Here the larvae and pupae live for many months. Protection is, therefore, afforded by building houses sited away from trees and by having dwellings wire-screened against the fly. Protective clothing and repellents are also useful. Mud flats where *Chrysops* is breeding should be treated with Dieldrin or other chemicals to destroy the larvae and pupae. Treatment of the population with diethylcarbamazine will diminish the infective rate of the potential vector.

Onchocerciasis

Onchocerciasis is the result of infection by the filaria *Onchocerca volvulus*. The adult female may be as long as 50 cm., the male being much shorter. The infection is conveyed by flies of the genus *Simulium* which inflict a painful bite. In West Africa the vector is *S. damnosum*, in Northern Nigeria also *S. bovis* and in East Africa and Congo *S. neavei*. The flies breed in rapidly flowing well aerated water, the larvae being attached to submerged vegetation and rocks. In the Congo and East Africa the larval flies may be attached to crabs and mayfly nymphs. Adult flies bite during the daytime both inside and outside houses. Man is the only known definitive host.

Geographical Distribution. Onchocerciasis occurs in well defined areas throughout tropical Africa, in Southern Arabia and also in South Mexico and Guatemala.

Pathology. Infective larvae of *O. volvulus* are introduced into the skin by the bite of an infected *Simulium*. In two to four months the worms mature. A group, including at least two intertwined living adult worms of different sexes, may become surrounded by fibrous tissue and a firm subcutaneous nodule results. The death of an adult worm may initiate the fibrosis. In these nodules, in the tissues around, and widely distributed in the skin, innumerable microfilariae, discharged by the female *O. volvulus*, move actively and may invade the anterior part of the eye. Although such microfilariae may be present with little tissue reaction, a severe dermatosis and similar tissue reactions in the eye may develop.

Clinical Features. No evidence of the infection, except for an eosinophilia, may be present for periods ranging from 9 to 24 months. The first sign may be the accidental discovery of one or more subcutaneous nodules, although the exploring hand is usually guided to their site by some degree of local irritation. Nodules are sometimes soft but more usually firm. They are subcutaneous but are sometimes attached to underlying bone or to overlying skin. Common sites are around the pelvis or around joints or the ribs and sometimes on the head. They vary in number and size and are painless. An additional or alternative and more common manifestation is a persistent irritating dermatosis, at first localised but gradually spreading and appearing also in multiple sites. In unpigmented skins this is seen as an erythematous rough maculopapular rash, often with excoriations following irresistible itching. In chronic infections the skin becomes inelastic, wrinkled and, in places, depigmented (leopard skin). Massive infiltration of the skin of the groin may cause it to hang down in a fold (hanging groin) and localised lymphatic obstruction may produce an elephantoid condition of the skin of the perineum.

In endemic areas the damage done to the eyes by microfilariae has earned the disease the name 'African River Blindness'. Lesions of the eye are more likely to be severe in areas of high endemicity. Early features are photophobia and conjunctival injection. The cornea may soon show interpalpebral 'snow-flake' deposits and later there may be ciliary injection, chronic iritis with adhesions, cyclitis and cataract. A mass of microfilariae in the anterior chamber may obstruct vision. Posterior segment changes of choroidoretinitis and optic atrophy have been described but it is doubtful if these lesions are usually due to onchocerciasis, nutritional or genetic factors being more likely in most cases.

Diagnosis. The finding of nodules or characteristic lesions of the skin or eyes, in a patient from an endemic area, associated with a considerable eosinophilia, is very suggestive of onchocerciasis. Aggravation of the dermatosis after treatment with diethylcarbamazine supports the diagnosis. A certain diagnosis may be made by removal of a nodule and the demonstration of adult worms and unsheathed microfilariae within it. A skin shaving, repeated if necessary from multiple sites, placed in warm saline or water and examined under the low power of the microscope, may reveal the microfilariae. They tend to migrate with gravity to the legs so that skin shavings should be taken initially from the loose skin below the lateral aspects of the knees or from the vicinity of a nodule. Microfilariae can also sometimes be seen moving in the anterior chamber of the eye examined with a slit-lamp or the $+20$ D lens of an ophthalmoscope or identified in a conjunctival biopsy. A filarial complement-fixation test is positive in about 50 per cent. of infections and the intradermal test in a much higher proportion. These are not specific for onchocerciasis (p. 88).

Treatment. Any nodules detected should be removed. Their removal, combined with a course of diethylcarbamazine, produces cure in a high percentage of cases.

Diethylcarbamazine (p. 89) rapidly kills the microfilariae and this causes an allergic reaction for the first few days of treatment. The itch increases, eye lesions are aggravated and there may be accompanying fever with pain in the joints. Only a small dose should be given initially, 0·5 mg./kg. body weight on the first day, this being gradually increased as the drug is tolerated until, if possible, a dose of 12 mg./kg. body weight is reached. This dose should be continued for 17 to 21 days. An antihistamine, such as chlorpheniramine maleate (Piriton) 4 mg. twice daily, will alleviate these allergic reactions and cortisone eye drops will control

the reaction in the eyes. The adult worm is more resistant to diethylcarbamazine and it is usually necessary to give two or more such courses
of treatment with it.

If repeated courses of diethylcarbamazine have failed to effect cure,
the more toxic drug suramin, which is more lethal to the adult worms,
should be employed, as in the treatment of trypanosomiasis (p. 10).
For onchocerciasis the intervals between intravenous injections of 1 g.
should be five to seven days and the maximum total dose 6 g. Besides
curing the dermatosis a surprising improvement of vision may result
from this treatment due to the removal of microfilariae which were
obstructing vision. If suramin alone fails to cure, a combination of oral
diethylcarbamazine and suramin, given intravenously, may succeed.

Prevention. Mass treatment of infected people with diethylcarbamazine
will reduce the infectivity of the vectors. The fly can be destroyed in its
larval stage by the application of Dieldrin to streams or the adult flies
can be attacked by spraying these insecticides on vegetation near streams.
Dimethylphthalate applied to skin or clothing will repel simulia for
several hours. Protective clothing should be worn round the legs to
discourage the fly from biting.

Dipetalonema streptocerca

Only the microfilariae of this parasite have been identified in man.
They have been found in the skin of man and chimpanzees. The microfilariae are unsheathed and are morphologically distinct from the microfilariae of *O. volvulus* and *D. perstans*. The intermediate host is *Culicoides
grahami*.

Geographical Distribution. Ghana and the Congo.

Clinical Features. The microfilariae may produce a mild dermatosis
of the trunk, usually less irritating than the dermatosis of onchocerciasis.

Diagnosis. The characteristic microfilariae may be found in skin
shavings (p. 93).

Treatment. A course of diethylcarbamazine as described for onchocerciasis is effective (p. 93).

Dipetalonema perstans

Dipetalonema (Acanthocheilonema) perstans is a filarial parasite of man
which is usually non-pathogenic. In endemic areas microfilariae of

D. perstans are commonly found in the peripheral blood. The adults inhabit chiefly the retroperitoneal and perirenal tissues and have been found in the pericardial sac. The microfilariae are unsheathed and do not exhibit any periodicity. The intermediate hosts are the small flies *Culicoides austeni* and *C. grahami*.

Geographical Distribution. This filaria is found throughout equatorial Africa as far south as Zambia, also in Trinidad and parts of Northern and Eastern South America.

Clinical Features. Sometimes it appears to be responsible for a persistent eosinophilia and perhaps occasional allergic manifestations. It has been suspected of causing effusions into serous cavities or a cardiomyopathy on rare occasions.

Treatment. *D. perstans* is relatively resistant to diethylcarbamazine and the infection may persist for many years.

Mansonella ozzardi

This filaria of man is non-pathogenic. The adults inhabit the mesentery and subperitoneal tissues. The microfilariae, which are unsheathed, circulate in the blood. The intermediate hosts are species of *Culicoides*.

Geographical Distribution. West Indies, Central and Northern parts of South America.

Clinical Features. None.

Treatment. None required. Diethylcarbamazine is ineffective.

Tropical Pulmonary Eosinophilia

Tropical pulmonary eosinophilia is a disease of uncertain aetiology. There are indications, however, that it may be caused by an infection with a filarial worm such as a *Dirofilaria* or *Brugia pahangi*, which is unable to mature in man. Alternatively it may be an unusual host reaction to *Wuchereria bancrofti* or *Brugia malayi*. Microfilariae have been demonstrated by liver and lung biopsy, and the filarial complement-fixation test (p. 88) has been found to be positive before treatment and negative after a course of diethylcarbamazine.

Geographical Distribution. The disease is found in many tropical regions including India, Ceylon, Malaysia, tropical Africa, China, Philippines, Australia and South America.

Pathology. Examination of lung tissue has revealed the presence of microfilariae surrounded by an eosinophilic cellular reaction and giant cells. Blood examination shows a leucocytosis, due to a great increase in the eosinophils.

Clinical Features. The illness commonly starts insidiously with cough, usually nocturnal and paroxysmal, accompanied by pains in the chest. Sputum is usually scanty but may be blood-stained. The cough often causes insomnia and may induce vomiting. There may be intervals of freedom from cough followed by recurrence of symptoms, often of increased severity with a rise of temperature. The patient's general health deteriorates and weakness and loss of weight may be marked. The most characteristic physical signs in the lungs are rhonchi and fine, medium or coarse crepitations. The expiration is usually prolonged but there is less bronchial spasm than in asthma. Sometimes, however, no abnormal physical signs are found in the lungs and in these cases the chief complaints may be tiredness and loss of weight. The most common radiographic finding is an increase in the normal lung striations, but miliary mottling is frequent; enlargement of the hilar glands is also common. Occasionally no abnormality is found in the lung on radiological examination. The eosinophil leucocyte count is always markedly increased. The erythrocyte sedimentation rate is raised up to 20 to 60 mm. in the first hour. Untreated the disease runs a prolonged non-fatal course with periods of remissions and exacerbations.

Diagnosis. The diagnosis is suggested by the symptoms and the associated raised leucocyte count of not less than 10,000/c.mm., of which at least 20 per cent. are eosinophils. Radiological examination of the chest may help, as also may a filarial complement-fixation test. In a patient suspected of suffering from this disease the rapid response to specific therapy supports the diagnosis. Pulmonary tuberculosis can be excluded by negative sputum tests and by the response to treatment. Other causes of eosinophilia such as bronchial asthma, Loeffler's syndrome, and the early stages of other helminthic infections such as schistosomiasis, and eosinophilic leukaemia have to be differentiated.

Treatment. Excellent results have been obtained with a short course of diethylcarbamazine. A dosage of 12 mg./kg. body weight daily in three divided doses for five days is usually adequate. With this treatment there is a rapid drop in the eosinophil count, the pulmonary features disappear and the patient's general health improves rapidly. A few relapse and require a further similar course of treatment.

DRACONTIASIS
(Guinea Worm Infection)

The female of the *Dracunculus medinensis* is a long thin nematode measuring a metre or more in length. It inhabits the interstitial and subcutaneous tissues of man and may produce an aseptic synovitis by penetrating a joint. The male is only 2·5 cm. long and dies early. The female lives from 12 to 18 months. The larvae are passed when the head of the gravid female breaks through the skin. After reaching water the larvae are taken up by a crustacean, *Cyclops* (water flea), in which they develop and become infective in about 21 days. The infected cyclops is found especially at the bottom of wells and ponds. When the cyclops is ingested by man the mature larvae penetrate the intestinal wall and migrate through the connective tissue of the host. After 9 to 18 months the fully mature female seeks the surface of the skin where a vesicle is raised, soon ruptures and exposes the anterior end of the worm. The distended uterus then ruptures and discharges its larvae externally. The worm is attracted to the surface by cooling, hence the larvae are likely to be expelled into water and to be ingested by a cyclops. Man is the most important host but *D. medinensis* has been found in dogs and cats.

Geographical Distribution. West, Central and East Africa, the Sudan, Arabia, Persia, Turkey, Pakistan, Central India, Burma, the Caribbean Islands and the northern parts of South America.

Clinical Features. When mature the adult may sometimes be felt beneath the skin. Some hours before the head of the worm emerges from the skin there is usually some local redness and tenderness. There may also be general allergic symptoms, erythema, giant urticaria, nausea, vomiting and diarrhoea. These symptoms usually subside as soon as the vesicle has ruptured and the larvae begin to be discharged. This is usually complete in three to four weeks, after which the worm is spontaneously extruded and healing takes place. The vesicle usually appears in the lower part of the leg or in any area which has been kept moist and relatively cool. If the worm dies or is broken during extraction there may be a marked reaction and bacterial infection may occur if pyogenic organisms are carried into the deep tissue by the retraction of the broken worm. Severe cellulitis, septicaemia, aseptic or pyogenic arthritis followed by contractions may result. Tetanus also is a well recognised complication.

Diagnosis. This is usually easy from the appearance of a vesicle and the recognition of the discharged larvae. A radiograph occasionally shows calcified worms.

Treatment. Diethylcarbamazine may destroy the immature female and hence should be used if infection is feared. Allergic features can be counteracted by adrenaline and antihistamine drugs. Niridazole (p. 75) is now successfully employed; the dose is 25 mg./kg. body weight daily in two divided doses for 10 days. Extraction of the worm, by winding it gently on a sterile orange-stick, is made easier and safer by the drug. Antibiotics and prophylaxis of tetanus may still be required in late cases with abscess formation.

Prevention. Water supplies should be protected against access of the larvae. This can be done by constructing a wall around the well, water then being drawn by means of a bucket. Cyclops may be destroyed by hyperchlorination, filtration or boiling of the water.

The co-operation of the community should be won by advising them as to the reasons for these preventive measures.

Diseases due to Fungi
(Mycotic Infections)

SUPERFICIAL MYCOSES

THE superficial mycoses affecting the skin are very common and occasionally the nails are affected.

Tinea versicolor (Syn. Pityriasis versicolor) is attributed to *Pityrosporum orbiculare* which produces fine scales of a yellowish or brown colour on the skin of the chest and abdomen. The sternal and interscapular regions are those most commonly affected. The discoloured areas spread at the periphery to give a fern-like appearance. There may be slight itching but the complaint is chiefly that of the disfigurement; the paler areas in a pigmented skin superficially resemble vitiligo or the hypopigmented lesions of leprosy. The absence of sensory changes and the fading margins distinguish the lesions from tuberculoid leprosy and the absence of *Myco. leprae* in skin slits and the demonstration of the fungus in potassium hydroxide preparations substantiates the morphological differences from lepromatous leprosy and seborrhoeic dermatitis. The lesions respond well to weak solutions of iodine, 20 per cent. sodium thiosulphate or to fungicidal ointments as recommended for dermatophytosis (see below) but there is a considerable likelihood of a relapse or re-infection.

Tinea imbricata, characterised by multiple concentric rings, is extremely common in coastal areas of some Pacific islands. It responds to griseofulvin (p. 100).

Dermatophytosis (ringworm infections) may be caused by a variety of fungi. According to the location of the lesion the condition may be described as tinea capitis, corporis, cruris or unguium when it affects the nails. The causative fungi may belong to the genera *Microsporum*, *Epidermophyton* or *Trichophyton*. On the body annular or serpiginous lesions with slight itching and no signs of leprosy usually create a characteristic picture, while between the toes the peeling sodden skin, sometimes associated with an unpleasant smell and inflamed surrounding tissues, is well known to doctors and to the lay public under the name of 'athlete's foot'. Infections of the nails are very persistent and cause them to be thickened, distorted and easily broken.

Sometimes in association with dermatophytosis of the feet there is an associated allergic erythematous dermatosis of the palms.

The diagnosis is confirmed by examining under the microscope small scales obtained by scraping the edge of the lesion. These are placed under a coverslip in warm 15 per cent. potassium hydroxide solution. The species is determined by culture on special media.

Whitfield's ointment containing salicylic acid and benzoic acid in equal parts in a base of soft paraffin and coconut oil is a long-established remedy and ointments containing undecylenate are also widely used. The fungicide now recommended is tolnaftate, 1 per cent. (Tinaderm). If there is much inflammation around the toes, the feet should be immersed in a solution of 1:10,000 potassium permanganate twice daily for several days until the reaction has subsided. Griseofulvin given without topical fungicides does not eradicate the fungi from the interdigital clefts but other resistant lesions, including infected finger nails, respond well to prolonged treatment with oral griseofulvin 250 mg. four times daily, although complete eradication especially from toe nails may take years to achieve. In the tropics, because of free perspiration, socks should be frequently washed and changed.

Tinea capitis in the tropics does not differ from that occurring in temperate climates. It is best treated by oral griseofulvin for three to five weeks.

Favus. Infection of the scalp by *Trichophyton schoenleinii* produces a mass of creamy white material with an offensive odour, the lesion being known as favus, or aptly in South Africa as witkop (white head). It is treated by epilation and powerful topical fungicides. When social conditions make prolonged oral therapy practicable griseofulvin has proved remarkably successful.

HISTOPLASMOSIS

Histoplasmosis is caused by *Histoplasma capsulatum* (*Darling*) which adopts a yeast-like morphology in its parasitic phase but is a filamentous fungus indigenous to soil at other times. A variant, *Histoplasma duboisii*, is found in parts of tropical Africa (p. 102). The spores of *Histoplasma* remain viable for years in the soil in which the fungus actually grows, and infected dust, when inhaled, conveys the disease. Occasionally infection passes through the buccal or intestinal mucosa or through the skin. The disease attacks dogs, rats and mice, and the fungus multiplies in soil enriched by the droppings of chickens, pigeons and bats. The infection is thus a hazard for explorers of caves.

Histoplasma capsulatum

Geographical Distribution. Histoplasmosis occurs in all parts of the United States of America, especially in the East Central States, and less commonly in Latin America from Mexico to Argentina, in Europe, North, South and East Africa, Nigeria, Malaysia, Indonesia and Australia.

Pathology. The parasite in its yeast phase multiplies like leishmaniae mainly in reticulo-endothelial cells but produces areas of necrosis in which the parasites may abound in enormous numbers. From these foci the blood stream may be invaded leading to enlargement of the liver, spleen and lymph nodes. Pulmonary histoplasmosis may produce pathological changes similar to those of tuberculosis (see below).

Clinical Features. Infection is usually carried to the lung in the first place by inhalation of dust containing spores. Probably 90 per cent. of pulmonary infections are benign producing no symptoms, but a more severe infection may closely simulate pulmonary tuberculosis, including the production of a primary complex with enlarged satellite lymph nodes, multiple small discrete lesions and occasionally cavity formation. Areas of calcification are characteristic of the more benign forms of this disease. Lesions of the skin or mucosa may be found on the rare occasions when infection has entered that way and are common in disseminated histoplasmosis which is characterised by enlargement of the liver, spleen and lymph nodes, irregular pyrexia, anaemia and leucopenia. An interesting feature is the frequency with which the adrenal glands become enlarged and caseous, producing symptoms of Addison's disease. Diseased heart valves, especially the aortic, are rarely invaded. When the mucosa of the mouth and gastrointestinal tract become infected, the predominant symptoms may be vomiting and diarrhoea. Occasionally the central nervous system is invaded. The severity of the symptoms of histoplasmosis varies from, in the majority of cases, a slight fever of short duration, like influenza, to a severe and prolonged pyrexial illness which ultimately proves fatal.

Diagnosis. In an area where the disease occurs, histoplasmosis should be suspected in every obscure infection in which there are pulmonary signs or where there are enlarged lymph nodes with or without hepatosplenomegaly. Material obtained by biopsy from a lymph node or the lung should be stained to show the intracellular *H. capsulatum*. It can also be demonstrated by culture or by animal inoculation. Radiological examination in old standing cases may show calcified lesions in the lungs, spleen or other organs. In the more acute phases of the disease single or multiple soft pulmonary shadows with enlarged tracheo-bronchial nodes may be revealed. An intradermal test is carried out with a 1:1000 dilution of a standardised histoplasmin antigen. This gives a positive reaction in most patients with either active or healed infections but is usually negative in the rapidly progressive form of the disease. A complement-fixation test is positive within three weeks of the onset of an acute primary histoplasmosis infection and increases in titre as the disease progresses. Precipitin tests are also employed.

Treatment. Rest and adequate diet are important. Sulphonamides are of limited value but amphotericin B is commonly used. This drug is primarily suppressive and is not free from serious side-effects. As amphotericin B is poorly absorbed from the intestine it has to be given intravenously. The dosage is 0·5 mg./kg. body weight, in 500 ml. of 5 per cent. glucose given over a six-hours period, gradually increasing to a maximum of 1·0 mg./kg. body weight. Daily treatment is necessary at first in seriously ill patients but later, as improvement sets in, it can be decreased to three times a week. If badly tolerated the dosage may have to be reduced. Side-effects are malaise, anorexia, nausea, fever and headache. These can be controlled to a considerable extent by the addition of 10 mg. prednisolone to the intravenous solution. Renal and hepatic function tests should be done during the course of treatment. Amphotericin B may have to be continued for up to a month or longer, depending on the clinical response. Recovery from generalised histoplasmosis is rare but recently a combination of trimethoprim and sulphamethoxazole (Septrin, Bactrim) has been used successfully.

Histoplasma duboisii

This fungus, first isolated in Ghana, is considerably larger than the classical *H. capsulatum*.

Geographical Distribution. Ghana, Uganda, Nigeria, Senegal, Sudan and the Congo.

Clinical Features. This disease differs in several ways from *H. capsulatum* infection. The bones, skin, lymph nodes and liver may be affected but the lungs are seldom involved. The visceral form with liver and splenic invasion is often fatal, while ulcerative skin lesions and bone abscesses follow a more benign course.

Radiological examination may show rounded foci of bone destruction sometimes associated with abscess formation. Multiple lesions of the ribs are common but the bones of the limbs may also be involved.

Treatment. The disease is treated in the same way as *H. capsulatum* infections. A solitary lesion in bone may require only local surgical treatment.

MYCETOMA
(Madura Foot)

In 1842 Gill of Madura in India described the condition which became known as Madura Foot. In 1860 Carter gave to this swelling, of fungal causation, the name 'mycetoma'. This clinical condition, which is not confined to infections of the foot, may be produced by members of two groups of organisms classified as *Maduromycetoma* and aerobic *Actino-myceteceae*. A feature common to both groups is the formation by the fungus of grains, with characteristic colours, ranging from 60 microns to 3 mm. in diameter. The incidence of different species appears to be related to climate, being especially high when an arid hot season ends in rains. The term 'mycetoma' is here used in this restricted sense, although some authors have used the term for other granulomatous lesions caused by fungi. The more common species of fungi causing mycetoma, as defined above, are:

Species	Type of Grains
Maduromycetoma	
Madurella mycetomi	brown or black (big)
Madurella grisea	black or brown (big)
Phialophora jeanselmei	black
Allescheria boydii	white or yellow (big)
Cephalosporium falciforme	white or yellow
Actinomycetecea	
Streptomyces madurae	white, yellow, red (big)
S. somaliensis	white or yellow (big)
S. pelletieri	red (small)
Nocardia caviae	yellow
Nocardia brasiliensis	white, yellow (very small)

The fungus can be identified by the microscopic appearances of the tissue and grains and confirmed by culture.

Nocardia asteroides closely resembles *N. caviae* but produces nocardi-osis, an infection in which grains are not produced.

Pathology and Clinical Features. The lesions may occur in any part of the body but as the fungus is probably usually introduced by a thorn they are most common in the foot and leg in peasants who walk bare-footed. At the site of implantation the mycetoma begins as a painless swelling, well localised in *Madurella mycetomi* infections. Unless totally excised at an early stage, or in some species effectively treated by chemo-therapy, the mycetoma grows and spreads inexorably and eventually penetrates local bones. The histology is that of a chronic granuloma with a fibrous stroma and cyst-like spaces in which lie the characteristic grains. The loose cellular tissue is infiltrated with leucocytes, small round cells and giant cells. Nodules develop under the epidermis and these rupture revealing sinuses through which mucopus containing the coloured grains is discharged. Some sinuses may heal with scarring while fresh sinuses appear elsewhere. There is little pain and usually no fever, but progressive disability. Secondary pyogenic infection does not usually penetrate far down the sinuses, possibly because of antibiotic activity of the fungi.

Madurella mycetomi grows in fascial planes and avoids the muscles until a very late stage; it does not affect nerves and tendons. Although pigment may be carried to regional lymph nodes, it is exceptional for the fungus to reach the nodes unless there has been surgical interference. When the lesion is in the scalp, the skull may be affected but the dura mater appears to be an effective barrier. Apart from involvement of bones by a spreading mycetoma, intra-osseous lesions may be found in the metaphysis of a long bone, especially at the upper end of the tibia and sometimes there may be an encapsulated periosteal mass.

Nocardia brasiliensis often affects the skin of the back. It is seldom localised and may spread widely.

Streptomyces somaliensis and *S. pelletieri* also spread insidiously and early invade muscle. As in the case of *S. madurae* they also readily reach regional lymph nodes.

Extensive damage of bones may be caused in any of these infections.

Treatment. The difference between *Maduromycetoma* and *Actinomycetecea* is crucial in that there is no drug of proven efficacy for the former. Amphotericin B is apparently inactive *in vivo*, though not necessarily *in vitro*, against both *Maduromycetoma* and aerobic actinomycetes that cause mycetoma. Sporadic successes with griseofulvin against the *Maduromycetoma* have been reported, but the results have been mostly disappointing. Experimental work is still going on with newer products like BAY b 5097 but up to the present maduromycetoma requires to be surgically removed. Mycetoma has a strong tendency to recur locally unless the excision has been adequate or the amputation high enough. The treatment of actinomycetoma is more hopeful. Dapsone frequently gives good results with infections due to *Nocardia* species. Sulphonamides also have some value. It is important to give the drug in an adequate dose for a long enough time. There are reports of the successful treatment of actinomycetoma due to *Streptomyces* species with dapsone, sulphonamides and broad spectrum antibiotics but there have also been many failures. Perhaps the most promising agent currently available for this group is a combination of trimethoprim and sulphamethoxazole (p. 102). Nevertheless, it must be admitted that many cases still require surgical removal.

NOTES ON OTHER MYCOSES

Blastomycoses

North American Blastomycosis is caused by *Blastomyces dermatitidis*. It also occurs in Africa. This infection may give rise to cutaneous lesions, especially of the face. Systemic infection begins in the lungs and mediastinal lymph nodes and resembles pulmonary tuberculosis. Bones, the central nervous system and the genito-urinary tract may also be affected.

Parenteral treatment with 2-hydroxystilbamidine (p. 4) or slow intravenous infusions of amphotericin B has achieved much success (p. 102).

South American Blastomycosis (*Paracoccidioidomycosis*) is caused by *Blastomyces brasiliensis*. Mucocutaneous lesions occur early. Involvement of lymphatic nodes and the lungs is prominent and the gastrointestinal tract may also be attacked.

Prolonged treatment with oral sulphonamides or slow intravenous infusions of amphotericin B may be curative. 2-hydroxystilbamidine may be successfully employed.

The diagnosis and differentiation of blastomycosis is established by culture of the fungus from the pus expressed from the lesion, or in systemic infections from the sputum. Complement-fixation reactions and intradermal tests aid diagnosis.

Chromoblastomycosis (Mossy Foot)

True mossy foot is a fungal infection and is to be distinguished from the warty excrescences which accompany the chronic lymphatic obstruction of elephantiasis and also from Madura Foot or mycetoma. Chromoblastomycosis is due to certain species of *Cladosporium*.

These fungi are acquired on splinters from decaying timber and give rise to a warty condition of the foot and also rarely affect the face, upper limbs, vulva and brain. The diagnosis is confirmed by the recognition of dark brown spheroid bodies 4 to 8 microns in diameter in biopsy specimens. These fungi grow readily on Sabouraud's medium.

Treatment. Iodides up to 3 g. daily and calciferol 1 to 2 mg. weekly should be given. This is combined, when necessary, with surgical removal of local lesions but relapse is common. Amphotericin B by 'blast' injection is now considered the best treatment.

Sporotrichosis

Sporotrichosis is caused by *Sporotrichum schenckii*. The infection occurs throughout the world and is prevalent in Central and Southern Africa. It causes swellings resembling gummata or a chancroid type of ulcer and affected lymphatic vessels may be thickened and palpable as a chain of nodules. Uncommonly dissemination takes place into lungs, bones, the central nervous system and elsewhere.

Diagnosis. The fungus can be cultured from discharges or biopsy material.

Treatment. Potassium iodide up to 10 g. daily should be given orally until some time after apparent clinical cure and into the lymph nodes a solution containing iodine in the proportions of 1 g. iodine, 10 g. potassium iodide in 500 ml. of water should be injected. Widely disseminated infections are successfully treated only by amphotericin B.

Cryptococcosis (Torulosis)

Cryptococcosis is caused by *Cryptococcus neoformans*. It occurs in India, California, Central United States and elsewhere and causes local gummatous-like tumours and granulomatous lesions of the lung, bones, brain and meninges. The cerebrospinal fluid often contains the fungus when the nervous system is affected.

Diagnosis. This is made by serological tests, biopsy or culture.

Treatment. Amphotericin B should be given by slow intravenous infusion and, in disease of the nervous system, intrathecally. It has been suggested from experimental work that a low thiamine diet and gamma globulin injections may be a useful supplementary measure. Some cases of cryptococcal meningitis have been cured by oral 5-fluorocytosine, 100 to 200 mg./kg. body weight given daily until the cerebrospinal fluid remained normal. Surgical removal of local pulmonary lesions is essential to prevent spread to the brain. Recovery may be assessed by serological changes.

Coccidioidomycosis

Coccidioidomycosis is caused by *Coccidioides immitis*. This infection is found in Southern United States, and in Central and South America. The disease is acquired by inhalation. In 40 per cent. of cases it affects the lungs and lymph nodes. Rarely it may be carried by the blood stream to the bones, adrenals, meninges and other organs. Infected sputum dribbling on to the chin produces a characteristic skin lesion. In 60 per cent. of cases the infection is asymptomatic. Infections, including subclinical attacks, are followed by immunity.

Diagnosis. The fungi appear as spherules, 11 to 70 micromicrons in diameter with a thick hyaline capsule containing numerous endospores. These grow readily on culture media but as they are highly infective, diagnostic investigations are usually limited to intradermal, complement-fixation and precipitin tests.

Treatment. Some localised pulmonary lesions can be successfully treated by surgery. The only treatment other than surgery which may be beneficial is the slow administration of intravenous infusions of amphotericin B.

Rhinosporidiosis

Rhinosporidiosis is caused by *Rhinosporidium seeberi* and occurs in South America, India, Ceylon, East Africa and elsewhere. This organism forms a cyst which on rupture discharges spores which spread by lymphatics to connective tissue. It produces polypi in the nose and localised swellings on the cheek and elsewhere.

Diagnosis. The characteristic sporangia and spores are recognised on histological examination of the tumour-like tissue but the organism has not yet been cultured.

Treatment. This consists of excision and intravenous pentavalent antimony (p. 3). Amphotericin B is required for resistant cases.

Miscellaneous Conditions

THE CHIGOE FLEA

INFESTATION with *Tunga penetrans* (the chigoe or jigger flea) is important in a number of tropical countries. Originally found in tropical America, it was introduced into Africa where it is widespread.

Clinical Features. The female *Tunga penetrans*, when impregnated, burrows into the skin of man, especially about the toes and soles, but the fingers and other parts of the body may be invaded. The flea then develops enormously, becomes as large as a pea and is packed with eggs in a cyst-like cavity. Ultimately the eggs are discharged on to the surface of the body. Man and pig are the principal hosts but cats, dogs, and rats may serve too. Untreated, the site of infestation may become irritated and inflamed but the chief danger is from secondary pyogenic infection. The anaerobic tissues around the chigoe are also suitable sites for the development of tetanus.

Treatment. An attempt should be made to remove the chigoe and egg sac complete but if it is ruptured no harm results if a mild antiseptic ointment is applied after removal of the chigoe and eggs. It is essential to avoid the introduction of bacteria by insisting on the use of a sterile needle when removing the chigoe. Massive infestations, such as may be seen in neglected children and in senile persons, should be treated by immersing the feet in a bath of an aqueous solution containing benzene hexachloride powder (BHC) 5 per cent. and Cetrimide powder 0·8 per cent.

Prophylaxis. The floor should be kept clean and sprayed with an insecticide. Shoes should be worn and the feet should be inspected daily, especially around the nails.

POROCEPHALOSIS

This name is given to invasions of the body by 'tongue worms', degenerate arthropods of which *Armillifer armillatus*, *A. moniliformis* and *Linguatula serrata* occur in man. Adult *Armillifer* parasitise the trachea and bronchi of snakes. Man is infected by ingesting ova on uncooked vegetables or by eating snakes. The condition is usually symptomless in man but calcified nymphs may be seen in radiographs of the chest and abdomen.

'Halzoun', the name given in the Middle East to acute dysphagia and laryngeal obstruction, due to pharyngitis and oedema of the larynx, following the eating of raw goats' liver was formerly attributed to invasion by immature *Fasciola hepatica* worms. It is now believed to be due to the ingestion of nymphs of *Linguatula serrata*. These may be obtained by eating the raw liver of goats or sheep but more commonly from the accompanying inadequately cooked lymph nodes of goats. Foxes and dogs are the definitive hosts and wild rodents or goats the intermediate hosts. Less commonly sheep are affected. Antihistamines and a local anaesthetic spray are suggested for treatment.

MYIASIS

Myiasis is an infestation of various tissues of man by the larvae of flies.

Cutaneous Myiasis

A common cause of cutaneous myiasis is *Cordylobia anthropophaga* (Tumbu fly). The larva penetrates the skin and produces a lesion like a boil. The eggs from which the larvae arise are liable to be laid on laundry spread on grass.

Another cause in the tropics is *Dermatobia hominis* which deposits its eggs on the ventral surface of the abdomen of other *Diptera*, especially mosquitoes. When the mosquito bites man or other animals, the warmth of the body stimulates the emergence of the larva. It burrows through the mosquito-made wound into the subcutaneous tissue and grows, causing a rounded swelling with a central orifice through which it obtains air. After reaching maturity it escapes. Occasionally the common warble fly (*Hypoderma bovis*) may infest man.

Auchmeromyia luteola, the Congo floor maggot, imbibes blood through the skin, dropping off when disturbed.

Treatment. The treatment of cutaneous myiasis consists of widening the opening in the skin, if necessary, and removing the larva.

Myiasis of Wounds, Sores and Cavities

The larvae of many flies including *Callitrogra hominivorax* (Screw worm), *Wohlfahrtia*, *Calliphora*, *Lucilia*, *Sarcophaga* and *Fannia* may infest necrotic tissue in open wounds or ulcers and occasionally invade living tissue. Chronic tropical ulcers and necrotic tissue from leprosy or tertiary yaws of the nose and pharynx may be invaded. *Chrysomia bezziana* is a myiasis-producing fly which is found in Africa, India and South Vietnam. It may penetrate the nasal sinuses and cause great tissue destruction. *Wolfahrtia magnifica* is the only specific myiasis-producing fly known to infest man in Europe.

Treatment. The application of 10 per cent. chloroform in a light vegetable oil is the treatment of choice for infested wounds.

Intestinal Myiasis

In the tropics especially, vague digestive disturbances or abdominal cramps with diarrhoea and vomiting may be caused by dipterous larvae in the intestinal canal. The eggs or larvae are ingested with food, but it is also possible for flies to deposit eggs on the skin around the anus whence the larvae may crawl into the rectum, vagina or even up the urethra and reach the bladder. Species of the genera *Fannia* and *Sarcophaga* are most frequently encountered. When larvae are swallowed they are passed in the stool or vomited. All fly larvae found in the stool have not necessarily been passed from the bowel as in tropical climates flies' eggs deposited in faecal matter rapidly hatch out into larvae. Occasionally larvae of *Aphiochaeta* or *Megaselia* may pupate in the bowel and live flies escape from the anus with the stool.

Treatment. An aperient is usually all that is required.

Aural Myiasis

When there is an aural discharge, myiasis may be caused by the larvae of *Callitrogra hominivorax*, *Sarcophaga*, *Calliphora* and *Fannia*. The nasal cavities and eyes may also be infested, and serious destruction may result.

Treatment. Instillation of 10 per cent. choloroform in a light oil kills the larvae.

Ocular Myiasis

The maggot of *Oestrus ovis* sometimes infests the human eye. The egg may be deposited in the eye of someone tending sheep, even without the fly alighting. A stinging sensation is felt, followed, as the larva develops, by severe pain in the eye. A drop of cocaine is required so that the lids can be opened to allow extraction of the maggot.

POISONOUS BITES

Snake Bite

Poisonous snakes belong to five families.

1. *Colubridae*, many of which are non-poisonous, include the Opistho-glypha which are poisonous but only rarely dangerous to man because

the grooved fangs are the most posterior teeth in the upper jaw. Examples are tree snakes.

2. *Elapidae* have forward grooved fangs. The fangs are fixed in the upper jaw below or in front of the eyes. The nostrils are lateral and there are large scales over the head. The family includes cobras, kraits and mambas.

3. *Hydrophidae* are poisonous sea-snakes; they have an eel-shaped tail and rather flattened body. Sea-snakes are found along the shores of the Indian and Pacific oceans and are mostly poisonous. The most common dangerous species is *Enhydrina schistosa*. *Laticauda colubrina*, the banded sea snake or 'coral snake' is poisonous but not aggressive.

The *Elapidae* and *Hydrophidae* both belong to the Proteroglypha, so named because the fangs lie anteriorly.

4. *Viperidae* are true vipers, including Russell viper and adders. At rest the long canalised fangs lie along the palate pointing posteriorly but during the act of biting are rotated forward.

5. *Crotalidae* include the pit viper (pit between the nose and the eye) and the rattlesnake.

The *Viperidae* and *Crotalidae* both belong to the Solenoglypha, the term indicating canalised fangs.

Snake venom is secreted as a specialised saliva from modified parotid glands. Its main function is to immobilise the prey but it appears also to assist in digestion. The venom may contain cellular debris and bacteria from the snake's mouth, e.g. *Cl. welchii*. The active agents in venom are enzymes which are antigenic; hence specific antisera can be prepared.

The amount of venom injected depends on various factors. A bite through clothing is less dangerous than one on the naked skin. The interposition of clothing makes a considerable difference to the bites of *Elapidae* as the fleshy covering of their grooved fangs is pushed aside and venom is lost on the surface of the skin, whereas the fully canalised fangs of the *Viperidae* enable venom to be discharged into the depths of the wound. Also the latter's poison glands are emptied ('wrung') more efficiently during the process of biting.

Pathology. The venoms of *Viperidae* and *Crotalidae* usually contain various powerful enzymes which are cytolytic and may also be haemolytic, cause haemorrhages or intravascular coagulation. The result is the production of a great swelling and necrosis of the tissues at the site of the bite.

The venom of the *Elapidae* is typically a powerful neurotoxic agent with only a slight cytolytic action, so producing very little local reaction. There are, however, important exceptions to this general statement, e.g. the Indian cobra. It is, therefore, prudent to acquire information about local poisonous snakes and the appropriate treatment for each so that the correct therapy may be made available.

Hydrophidae secrete a potent venom containing a myotoxin which produces necrosis of muscles.

Clinical Features. The bites of *Viperidae* and *Crotalidae* are characterised by a profound local effect on the tissues at the site of the wound. Severe pain, great swelling and discoloration from haemorrhage and oozing of blood-stained serum are usually followed by sloughing. General symptoms, when pronounced, are those of cardiovascular shock accompanied by nausea and vomiting. If the venom has gained access to a vein, the victim may die in a few minutes from massive intravascular clotting. When, more commonly, the venom is injected extravenously, the patient may die of cardiac failure associated with severe anaemia. Local sloughing is often complicated by secondary sepsis and may be followed by gas gangrene or tetanus.

Elapine bites may show few local signs apart from some numbness and some early muscular weakness. Within two hours there follows the sequence of drooping eyelids, unsteady gait, incoordinate speech and difficulty in respiration. Later general and bulbar paralysis develop, with difficulty in swallowing, aphasia and cyanosis. The heart is not primarily affected, and consciousness is retained until near the end. Death may come within six hours or be delayed for one or two days.

Fishermen dragging nets ashore in muddy water, at or near a river mouth, are the usual victims of bites by *Hydrophidae*. Bathers and paddlers are seldom attacked. The bite on ankle, foot, wrist or hand is felt as a sharp prick but thereafter is painless, inconspicuous and without local swelling. Systemic poisoning follows in only a quarter of those bitten. In these, symptoms appear within one hour and consist of pain and stiffness, initially in the muscles of the neck, back and proximal parts of the limbs but rapidly becoming generalised. Passive movements provoke intense pain. Later, in severe poisoning, trismus, ptosis and external ophthalmoplegia may appear. Three to six hours after the onset of poisoning, the urine contains myoglobin and protein. Death may result from extensive paresis leading to respiratory failure or from renal failure. If poisoning is less severe, the victim survives but muscle weakness may persist for months.

Treatment. The following first-aid measures can be carried out by untrained personnel. First determine, if possible, whether the bite is of a poisonous snake by examining and retaining the snake, if available, and by searching the bite for fang punctures. As most people bitten by a snake suffer from fright and fear of death the patient must be reassured that fatal results from snake-bite are uncommon. The patient must be kept at rest and a constricting ligature such as a handkerchief applied above the wound sufficiently firmly to retard the flow in the veins and lymphatics draining the bitten area but not to stop the arterial circulation. The ligature must be released for one minute in every thirty. Venom on the surface of the wound should be wiped away gently with a cloth or washed away with plain water. The bitten part should be immobilised as for a fracture and an analgesic such as aspirin but not morphia may be given. Medical aid should be obtained as soon as possible.

The further treatment depends on the type of venomous snake.

In Great Britain *Vipera berus* is the only poisonous snake, and its bite is less dangerous than is the use of antivenom. The only antivenom available is that prepared for use against *Cerastes cornutus*, a South African viper, and its efficacy against *Vipera berus* is unproved and its use is not recommended. As soon as medical care is available, the further treatment of a viper bite in Britain is the injection of 100 mg. hydrocortisone intramuscularly, 1 to 2 mega units of penicillin and a 'recall' dose of tetanus toxoid or, in the unprotected, 2,000 units of tetanus antitoxin. The lightly applied tourniquet will subsequently be released with increased frequency.

In countries where a highly venomous land snake may have bitten a person, further treatment as discussed below can be given by non-medically qualified persons who have had first-aid training. Specific or polyvalent antivenom 10 to 30 ml. may be given by the intramuscular route using one or more sites of injection. The dose of antivenom must be repeated after four hours. It should be remembered that a child requires as large a dose of antivenom as an adult. At the same time, to lessen the risk of anaphylaxis, 1 ml. of adrenaline injection B.P. should be given slowly intramuscularly and half this dose can be repeated 15 minutes later. Prednisolone 30 mg. is given by mouth or hydrocortisone hemisuccinate 100 mg. intramuscularly. Ice bags are applied to the bitten part, which, however, must not be immersed in ice or ice-cold water. Penicillin and anti-tetanus treatment are given as well.

When a doctor is available the same treatment is recommended but the antivenom should be given in the same dosage by the intravenous route. Except in extreme urgency it is advisable to give a trial dose of 0·2 ml. antivenom intramuscularly and to observe the patient for 30 or preferably 60 minutes for signs of anaphylaxis before the therapeutic dose is injected intravenously. The intramuscular route may be used for children with small veins. Incision into the swollen part is indicated only when there is marked swelling likely to cause gangrene, and this should be undertaken only by a medical man.

Those bitten by sea-snakes should be given similar first-aid treatment, being kept at rest and transported by stretcher to hospital. If more than one hour elapses after the bite without the appearance of signs of toxicity only reassurance is required. If there is clear evidence of systemic poisoning specific anti-serum should be given intravenously, preferably after testing for anaphylaxis. A dose of 2 to 3 ampoules is advised but this should be increased to 4 or 5 ampoules if signs of severe systemic poisoning are present.

GENERAL MEASURES. Shock should be combated by rest, warmth and fluid by mouth or intravenously, and blood should be transfused when indicated. To control haemorrhage calcium salts and vitamin K may be useful. Respiratory weakness following an elapine bite will benefit from oxygen and respiratory paralysis by mouth-to-mouth breathing or by the intratracheal method. Bacterial infection is more likely in *Viperidae* and *Crotalidae* bites, and here penicillin, tetanus toxoid or antitoxin and anti-gas gangrene serum are especially useful.

Spider Bite

The venom of certain spiders is dangerous to man. One of them is *Latrodectus mactans*, the 'black widow' spider. The adult female is glossy-black with crimson hour-glass markings on the ventral aspect of the abdomen. In South Africa *L. indistinctus*, the 'button' spider, is also poisonous as is *Atrax robustus*, the 'funeral web' spider, in Australia. Many other poisonous arachnids are found in different parts of the world. With the bite venom is injected and this causes severe local pain followed by redness and swelling. Soon pain is intense, first in the adjacent muscles but spreading rapidly to all voluntary muscles, especially the flexor groups, causing severe spasms. Contraction of the pupils, salivation and sweating are common, and in severe cases the patient may suffer cardiovascular collapse. Rigidity of the abdominal muscles may simulate an acute abdomen. Later the site of the bite may slough.

Treatment. The bite should be cleansed. Local incision and suction may remove some of the venom. Where a specific antivenom is available this should be injected into the muscles near the bite. If convalescent serum is available it may be tried. A good response may be obtained to an injection of atropine. Corticosteroids are of value. For the relief of muscle spasm 10 to 20 ml. of 10 per cent. calcium gluconate can be given slowly intravenously. Antibiotics should be used against secondary pyogenic infections.

Octopus Bite

The octopus seizes its prey by its eight tentacles and inflicts a painful bite which is not, however, usually dangerous.

Tick Paralysis

Animals and occasionally man suffer from fatal poisoning due to venom excreted by the salivary glands of certain *Ixodidae* (hard ticks). This is especially likely to follow the attachment of the tick to the head or neck for some days. A flaccid paralysis may develop followed by failure of respiration. Removal of the tick, in time, leads to recovery.

POISONOUS STINGS

Scorpions

There are many genera of scorpions found in the tropics and subtropics. Paired poison glands are situated in the terminal segment of the flexible jointed tail which is curved dorsally over the scorpion's body before striking.

Clinical Features. There is a single puncture wound at the site of the sting. Intense local pain is felt immediately, and a red oedematous wheal, sometimes haemorrhagic, soon appears. Children particularly show severe general symptoms which include sweating, salivation, nausea, vomiting and depression of respiration and may die. From S. India and Jordan occasional deaths of adults also are reported and recent observations point to disseminated intravascular coagulation resulting in defibrination and haemorrhages as the cause of death. In Trinidad stings of the scorpion *Tityus trinitatis* frequently cause acute pancreatitis from which recovery is usual.

Treatment. Pain can be relieved by applications of ice-cold water or by the local injection of xylocaine and adrenaline. When a young child has been stung, the site of the sting should be cleansed with soap and water and incised. Local suction is then of value in removing some of the venom. If antivenom is available the child should be given 5 ml. of the serum intramuscularly near the sting as early as possible. When required, general treatment for shock is given. The value of corticosteroids is under investigation and in severe cases continuous intravenous heparin would combat disseminated intravascular coagulation.

Bee Stings

A bee sting is always painful and in those who have become sensitised an anaphylactic reaction may result in rapid death. In the majority of fatal cases there has been a severe reaction to a bee sting on an earlier occasion. Desensitisation may be practised with some degree of success. Emergency treatment of anaphylactic shock consists of the intramuscular injection of 0·5 ml. of adrenaline solution followed by an intravenous injection of hydrocortisone hemisuccinate 100 mg. Anyone who has sustained a severe reaction should, however, be furnished with the means of self-administering a subcutaneous injection of 0·5 ml. of adrenaline solution in an emergency and should also carry a drug such as isoprenaline, 10 mg. of which placed under the tongue produces rapid stimulation of the sympathetic nervous system. Less severe symptoms may be relieved by an antihistamine. Multiple stings are more dangerous than single stings and the 'stingers' of the bees should be removed from the skin as they continue to release venom until this has been done.

Jellyfish

Various jellyfishes cause lesions in the skin and general reactions in man. Stinging by the Portuguese man-of-war, *Physalia*, is commonly associated with these reactions. The long filamentous tentacles hanging from its under surface contain poison glands which release a toxin when they come in contact with the human skin. Linear reddish-brown wheals are produced in the affected areas of skin. Excruciating local pain is felt, and soon general symptoms may follow, including profuse sweating and severe griping abdominal pains. Very occasionally a patient dies within a short time of being stung by a jellyfish, in which case one of the *Cubomedusae* (sea-wasps or box-jellies), *Chironex fleckeri* or *Chiropsalmus quadrigatus* is probably responsible. Their tentacles contain numerous characteristic stinging organs which have been identified in the lesions of those who have succumbed. The stings are very painful. At postmortem the lungs and air passages have been filled with frothy mucus and the abdominal organs and brain are congested. 'Irukandji stings' affect bathers in the sea off N.E. Australia at certain seasons. They are caused by minute Carybdeid (simple sea-wasps). Acute poisoning develops in a few minutes characterised by violent abdominal and generalised pains, vomiting and prostration. The victim appears seriously ill for a few days but always recovers.

Treatment. The exact nature of the poison is not known but in severe cases the intramuscular injection of an antihistamine drug should be employed without delay. Corticosteroids may also be of value. The stinging organs may adhere to cellophane tape applied over the affected area and be withdrawn when this is removed. A cream or ointment should not be applied as this spreads the affection.

Cone Shells (Conidae)

There are many varieties of cone shells. The occupant is often poisonous and can give a sting causing death by respiratory paralysis.

Stinging Fish

The stonefish (*Synanceja trachynis*) is the most deadly of the stinging fish and it can easily be mistaken for a piece of coral. Along its back are 13 large spines each containing paired poison sacks. The poison causes great pain and swelling at the sites of the stings and may cause death from respiratory paralysis. Hot water destroys the poison and an antivenom is available.

The stingrays (*Dasyatidae*) are flat fish lying on the sand or mud. When disturbed a painful sting may be inflicted from a poisonous spine of the tail.

Poisonous Fish

There are a number of fish which may be poisonous to eat. Examples are the pufferfish (*Tetraodontidae*), porcupine fish (*Diodontidae*) and box-fish (*Ostraciontidae*). In general, fish covered with hard plates or spines may be poisonous, and the skin and liver, in particular, are dangerous to eat.

TROPICAL PHLEBITIS

This phlebitis, of uncertain origin, was first described in East Africa but is now known to occur throughout tropical Africa.

Pathology. Vascular granulation tissue containing fibroblasts, endothelial cells and giant cells is laid down, especially in the middle coat of the vein but extends outside the wall of the vein. Thrombosis takes place in the vicinity of the lesion and distal to it. Thrombosis of the splenic vein may cause necrotic infarction and liquefaction in the spleen.

Clinical Features. The effect of these changes in a vein depends on its size. When the vein is large, there will be a marked reaction in it with pain along its course, followed by local swelling and enlargement of the veins and tissues distal to the lesion. It may be possible to palpate the affected vein as a hard cord-like structure. There is usually a febrile reaction during the acute stage. The venous lesion gradually resolves and the circulation is re-established. When the diseased veins are small, the symptoms and signs are slighter. Painful thickenings of one or several superficial veins may be palpated. These usually resolve in a few weeks.

Diagnosis. This is made by a history of local pain over a vein, with swelling and constitutional disturbance. When one of the larger veins is affected, the initial symptoms may resemble those of tropical myositis. Meningitis may be simulated by phlebitis of veins in the neck.

Treatment. This is symptomatic. The value of treatment with anti-coagulants has not been determined.

TROPICAL MYOSITIS
(Pyomyositis)

The cause of myositis in the tropics is uncertain. If explored early no bacteria are found but later the pus contains staphylococci or streptococci. The disease usually occurs in malnourished persons. It has been thought that in some instances 'tropical phlebitis' may precede the myositis but pyomyositis occurs frequently in New Guinea where tropical phlebitis is not encountered.

Geographical Distribution. Most cases occur in tropical Africa, South America and South Pacific Islands.

Clinical Features. Pyomyositis starts with fever and induration of one or more of the large muscles, mostly in the lower limbs. The indurated area subsequently suppurates and a large abscess may form and be associated with a swinging temperature and leucocytosis. The affected area is swollen, hot and tender. When the pus is superficial, fluctuation can be detected.

Diagnosis. This is usually not difficult except when the psoas muscle is involved. The differential diagnosis includes Calabar swellings, scurvy and an underlying osteomyelitis. Staphylococcal pyaemia of other origin is characterised by numerous small abscesses. *Diphyllobothrium mansoni* in the larval stage, known as a sparganum, may be found in an abscess in the muscles in some endemic regions.

Treatment. The patient should be nursed in bed. When an abscess has formed, it should be aspirated and a suitable antibiotic given, but if resolution is delayed the abscess must be incised and the pus evacuated.

CIRRHOSIS OF THE LIVER PECULIAR
TO THE TROPICS

Cirrhosis of the liver is frequent in underdeveloped countries where malnutrition prevails and it appeared probable that a relative and absolute deficiency of protein led to the cirrhosis either directly or indirectly by predisposing the liver to noxious agents such as toxins, parasites and viruses. It is now thought that dietary deficiencies may only have a secondary role. Hepatotoxins, in herbs or contaminating foodstuffs, of the pyrrolizidine group have been isolated as retrorsine and mono-crotaline. Pyrrolizidine alkaloids have been shown, experimentally in animals, to produce cirrhosis and hepatoma. Aflatoxins isolated from fungi contaminating grain used for feeding animals have also caused cirrhosis and hepatoma experimentally. Infective hepatitis (p. **635**) is very common in the tropics. Cirrhosis of the liver or lesser degrees of fibrosis may also arise in the conditions described below.

Veno-occlusive Disease of the Liver

This disorder has been reported chiefly from Jamaica but it extends beyond the West Indies and has been described in South Africa. The disease affects persons of all ages but most frequently children from 2 to 5 years of age. Its aetiology is still uncertain, but there is evidence that a poison in 'bush tea' infused from plants, *Senecio* (ragwort) and *Crotalaria*, causes the disease in malnourished children. Animals injected with extracts from these plants have developed similar changes in the liver.

Pathology. The acute stage of the disease shows occlusion of the centrilobular veins by proliferation of the intimal cells and swelling of the subintimal tissue. This leads to back pressure atrophy of the liver cells and, if the patient survives for some time, centrilobular fibrosis.

Clinical Features. The disease may occur in an acute form with rapid enlargement of the liver and ascites but usually without jaundice and splenomegaly; death from hepatic failure may follow after a few days. However, with or without treatment, complete recovery is possible, or a subacute stage, with enlargement of the liver but few symptoms of ill-health, may ensue. From this the patient may gradually recover or the fibrosis may progress so that the liver becomes extensively cirrhotic with all the symptoms and signs of portal hypertension and hepatic failure.

Treatment. A well balanced diet with adequate animal protein must be given and all forms of 'bush tea' excluded.

Indian Childhood Cirrhosis

This disease occurs in the children of strict vegetarians in India. The children are not obviously malnourished, the majority being breast-fed and not belonging to the poorest families. The incidence is predominantly in males between 1 and 3 years of age. As more than one case occurs in over 50 per cent. of affected families, a sex linked genetic factor appears probable. There is no evidence of a dietary toxin. A defect of cellular ability to deal with the virus of infective hepatitis has been postulated.

E

Pathology. There is diffuse necrosis of liver cells with replacement fibrosis. The degenerate cells appear as granular and smudged eosinophilic masses. Fibrosis is of portal type involving small groups of cells with complete loss of normal hepatic architecture. The veins are unaffected.

Clinical Features. The disease may be fulminating, acute with death within one to three months, or subacute nearly always proving fatal within one year. Enlargement of the liver is invariable and is accompanied in the majority by splenomegaly, ascites and jaundice.

Treatment. This should be on the same lines as for infective hepatitis (p. 645).

Iron and Cirrhosis of the Liver

(Bantu Siderosis)

Hepatic cirrhosis associated with siderosis has been found amongst the adult Bantu of South Africa as well as in Ghana. The large amounts of haemosiderin in the body are thought to be due to the high intake of iron acquired through preparing food and beer in iron vessels. Some consider that excessive iron storage is more likely to be the result of abnormal liver cell metabolism due to protein malnutrition or to a fault in the intestinal barrier against excessive iron intake. A somewhat similar liver cirrhosis is found in Bantu porphyria; the cause here may also be a toxic factor in impure beer.

Pathology. Haemosiderin is deposited in the tissues of the body, including the liver, where it may set up a reactionary fibrosis ending in cirrhosis. Osteoporosis, associated with a vascular necrosis of the head of the femur is frequent.

Malaria

Chronic malaria may cause a reaction in the liver with fibrous tissue formation limited to the periportal region. However, in certain hyperendemic areas of malaria sufferers from a severe degree of malnutrition and malaria have been found to have a diffuse fibrosis of the liver.

Brucellosis

In brucellosis granulomatous deposits occur in the liver and other organs, but only rarely has cirrhosis of the liver been seen to develop in the absence of other aetiological factors.

Sickle-cell Anaemia

In sickle-cell anaemia the liver is often altered in structure and function as a result of the combined effect of anaemia, capillary obstruction by masses of sickle cells and distension of Kupffer cells with phagocytosed erythrocytes. Focal necrosis, scarring and fibrosis of the liver are therefore often found in sickle-cell anaemia (p. 147).

Helminthic Infections

Fibrosis of the liver in association with schistosomiasis (p. 72), clonorchiasis (p. 76) and fascioliasis (p. 79) is well recognised.

TROPICAL ULCER

The aetiology of tropical ulcers is still in doubt. Predisposing factors are dysentery, minor injuries occurring in the presence of undernourishment, poor hygienic surroundings and debilitating diseases such as malaria. The bacillus *Fusobacterium fusiforme* and the spirochaete *Borrelia vincenti* can usually be demonstrated in the ulcer, but the part they play in its production is uncertain. Experimentally, discharge from an active lesion kept in contact with damaged tissue has reproduced the ulcer in man. The disease is widely distributed in tropical countries, occasionally in epidemic form, particularly after a famine.

Pathology. The edges of the ulcer are raised, thick, oedematous and infiltrated with neutrophils. In the early stages the ulcerated area is covered with necrotic skin, and the underlying tissue shows fibroblastic proliferation. Very severe cases may show destruction down to the periosteum. Staphylococci and streptococci are usually present in addition to *F. fusiforme* and *Bor. vincenti*.

Clinical Features. The initial lesion of a tropical ulcer is a bleb filled with sanguineous fluid. It may be painful and itchy with some constitutional upset. Soon the bleb ruptures, and a green-grey moist slough is exposed which rapidly spreads in the skin and subcutaneous tissue up to a diameter of 5 cm. or more. In a few days these tissues slough and liquefy releasing a very offensive discharge. Further extension may take place peripherally. After a week or more there is usually no further spread and the necrotic tissue separates, exposing an ulcer which remains more or less stationary. In the chronic state the edges of the ulcer are raised and slope down sharply towards the ulcerated surface. The damage may be limited to the skin and superficial fascia, but in severe cases deep structures, e.g. tendons, nerves, blood vessels and periosteum, may be invaded. Bone is rarely affected (although the ulcer over a sequestrum of chronic osteomyelitis may simulate a tropical ulcer). Tropical ulcers generally affect the parts of the body exposed to trauma, especially the lower third of the leg and the foot. The ulcer is usually solitary, but after healing no immunity is developed against a recurrence.

General constitutional effects of a tropical ulcer are slight, and adenitis is not found except as a result of secondary infection.

The ulcer heals slowly with a tissue-paper-like scar which may break down from very slight trauma. When the lesion has been severe enough to destroy deeper tissues, scarring and deformity result; if near a joint it may cause ankylosis. Carcinoma (epithelioma) sometimes arises in the edge of a very chronic tropical ulcer. These growths are usually of relatively low malignancy. In regions where neglected tropical ulcers are frequent they constitute one of the more common causes of malignancy.

Diagnosis. The appearance and progress of an ulcer with few constitutional symptoms are characteristic. Isolation of *Bor. vincenti* and *F. fusiforme* is confirmatory. Early cutaneous diphtheria may be mistaken for a tropical ulcer, but constitutional symptoms are severe and *Cl. diphtheriae* may be isolated. A chronic ulcer of yaws or syphilis will be associated with a positive Wassermann reaction and perhaps other signs of a treponematosis. Buruli ulcer is described below.

Treatment. Rest in bed with elevation of the affected part and a generous diet with adequate proteins are important. Local treatment consists in thorough cleansing of the ulcer with hypertonic magnesium sulphate. Penicillin as PAM (300,000 units) intramuscularly, repeated in 48 hours, or tetracycline 2 g. daily for seven days gives good results. In very chronic cases, after cleansing and treatment with antibiotics, excision of the ulcer and scar tissue may be required, to be followed by skin grafting.

Ambulant treatment, with the ulcerative area supported with strips of adhesive plaster, may be effective when rest cannot be enforced. The dressing is changed at intervals of about five days. Antibiotics should be given.

Prophylaxis. Where tropical ulcers are a risk, abrasions should be cleansed and covered without delay. The provision of a good diet, washing facilities and a first-aid service has abolished tropical ulcers from labour forces on well-run estates in the tropics.

BURULI ULCER

This condition, first accurately described in Australia and New Guinea but named from its frequency in Buruli in the Nile valley of Uganda, is caused by the acid-fast organism, *Mycobacterium ulcerans*. The epidemiology is unknown but all the known foci of infection are near to rivers of considerable size. It is now recognised to begin usually as a single small subcutaneous nodule situated commonly on the leg or forearm. The skin over the centre of the nodule ulcerates and, untreated, the ulcer extends to involve a progressively large area. Histologically there is much necrosis of subcutaneous fat and *Myco. ulcerans* are abundant in the necrotic tissue in the base of the ulcer.

If suspected before ulceration, the nodule should be excised when healing readily occurs. Ulcers require to be excised and skin grafted. In addition drugs effective in the treatment of leprosy have been employed, the most promising being clofazimine (p. 25).

BURKITT'S LYMPHOMA

Since the original description by D. P. Burkitt in Uganda in 1958 there has been increasing interest in this particular form of malignant lymphoma, now recognised as the most common neoplasm affecting children in certain parts of tropical Africa. The tumour has also been described from many other countries.

Aetiology. In view of the demonstrated relationship between the incidence of this tumour and climatic factors of temperature and rainfall, it was assumed that some biological agent must be implicated. Since the geographical distribution of the tumour corresponds to that of several insect vectors it was postulated that an arbovirus might be the causative agent. The subsequent recognition that large areas of the moist tropics were free from this tumour necessitated a modification of this concept, and it is now postulated that the high incidence in certain areas may be the result of changes in the lymphoreticular system caused by persistent malaria. It is suggested that an ubiquitous virus, possibly the Epstein-Barr virus, evidence of which can be found in all patients with this tumour, tends to produce neoplastic change more frequently when acting on cells already altered by chronic malaria.

Pathology. Extensive studies have shown that this tumour is a malignant lymphoma of poorly differentiated lymphoblastic type. The histological pattern is of uniform masses of immature lymphoid cells. Interspersed between these cells are many large clear histiocytes with poorly staining cytoplasm which may contain cell debris. The so-called 'starry sky' pattern seen in sections of the tumour is due to these large histiocytes. Cellular detail is more easily seen and interpreted in the stained imprint preparations from fresh unfixed tissues, than in ordinary histological sections.

Clinical Features. In Africa this tumour has a peak incidence between the ages of 4 and 8 years. Relatively few cases occur after puberty, but occasional cases are seen in adult life. The most frequent presenting feature is a tumour of the mandible or maxilla. The first clinical sign is usually loosening of the molar and pre-molar teeth which eventually become displaced, distorted and lost as the tumour grows. Tumours of the maxilla may present as exophthalmos due to early invasion of the orbit. The eye may eventually be totally destroyed and at this stage it is difficult to distinguish this tumour from a retinoblastoma. A particularly characteristic feature is the tendency for the tumours in the jaws to be multiple and it is not uncommon for all four jaw quadrants to be involved simultaneously.

The second commonest clinical presentation is an abdominal tumour, usually caused by involvement of the kidneys, adrenals, ovaries, liver or abdominal lymph nodes. Involvement of the kidneys, adrenals and ovaries is often bilateral.

The third commonest presenting feature is paraplegia which is of sudden onset, flaccid from the outset and associated with incontinence of urine and faeces, without radiological evidence of vertebral collapse.

Other sites characteristically involved in this multifocal tumour are the long bones of the limbs, the thyroid and salivary glands, the testes and the heart. Bilateral massive tumours of the breasts sometimes develop in young adult women.

The rarity of peripheral lymphadenopathy is particularly characteristic.

Treatment. This tumour is unusually sensitive to a large range of cytotoxic drugs and to radiotherapy. As the tumour is probably always multifocal, systemic chemotherapy is preferred. The best results to date have been obtained with cyclophosphamide and orthomerphalan. The former is given in single large doses of 30 to 40 mg./kg. body weight repeated on one or more occasions after recovery of marrow depression. The latter is given in one or two doses of 1·1 to 1·4 mg./kg. A more extensive regime using multiple drugs has been used with success in resistant tumours. Intracranial involvement, recognised by the presence of tumour cells in the C.S.F., should be treated with methotrexate. In some clinics in Africa prolonged survival rates of over 30 per cent. have been reported.

IDIOPATHIC MULTIPLE HAEMORRHAGIC SARCOMA OF THE SKIN
(Kaposi's Sarcoma)

This strange multiple neoplasm in skin, first described in Europe in 1872, which is rare in Europe and America, is now known to be relatively common in many parts of Africa. It predominantly affects men. The aetiology and the reasons for its geographical distribution and sex and age incidence are unknown.

Pathology. The tumours of the skin are well defined nodules which consist of new blood vessels and large spindle cells with numerous mitotic figures. Pigment granules free in the tissue or within histiocytes are easily seen. Strands of connective tissue, infiltrated with plasma cells and lymphocytes, run through the nodule. The peripheral lymphatics are often markedly dilated. At autopsy visceral lesions can be demonstrated in almost all tissues except the brain but rarely give rise to symptoms.

Clinical Features. Vague paraesthesiae, local sweating or oedema may precede the appearance of nodules in a proportion of cases but the appearance of a nodule in the skin of one limb is the first important diagnostic feature. The nodules vary in size from 2 to 20 mm. in diameter. They are blue or brown in colour, firm and elastic to touch and have a smooth surface. The appearance is highly characteristic. They may coalesce, ulcerate and become infected, followed by overgrowth of granulation tissue. In order of decreasing frequency nodules occur in the skin of the feet, legs, hands, arms, trunk, genitalia, head and neck.

Lymph nodes are enlarged in half the cases but they are not usually invaded by the tumour. Oedema is common, varying from slight local swelling to gross enlargement of a whole limb. The latter indicates involvement of the deeper soft tissues and bone.

A unique feature is spontaneous regression and complete disappearance of individual nodules although the disease as a whole may be progressing.

Diagnosis. The condition is suspected from the striking clinical picture and biopsy reveals the characteristic histology. Radiological studies by soft tissue films may show unsuspected nodules throughout an affected limb, and bony lesions are demonstrated as generalised or localised rarefaction, loss of trabeculation, cortical erosion or cysts.

Prognosis. The condition is slowly progressive and ultimately fatal in an average time of eight years, but occasionally the course is rapid and fulminating.

Treatment. The tumours, although radiosensitive, may be too widespread for effective radiotherapy. High voltage therapy throughout the depth of a limb is usually required, since superficial irradiation is only of value for the early superficial nodules. As radiotherapy is not available in many parts of Africa and surgery can offer only limited benefits, chemotherapy is the treatment of choice.

Intra-arterial regional perfusion of the limb or limbs with nitrogen mustard or other cytotoxic drugs has caused improvement in a proportion of cases. Regression of the disease may be prolonged by the oral administration of 0·5 mg. of triaziquone twice a week. These effects are however only transient and palliative in the more severe and malignant forms of the disease.

EPIDEMIC DROPSY

(Argemone Poisoning)

This disease is due to the use of mustard oil contaminated with the seeds of a poppy weed, *Argemone mexicana*. The weed grows commonly in mustard crops and contains a toxic alkaloid, sanguinarine. This substance interferes with the oxidation of pyruvic acid, which accumulates in the blood and tissues of the patient. Epidemic dropsy occurs in groups of people partaking of the same food, especially curried rice prepared with contaminated mustard oil.

Geographical Distribution. Epidemic dropsy is encountered in India, especially in Bengal, Bihar, Orissa, Madhya Pradesh and Uttar Pradesh. Cases have also been noted among Indian expatriates in Fiji.

Pathology. There is general dilatation of the smaller arterioles and of the capillaries, especially those of the skin, heart muscle and uveal tract. New blood vessels in the deeper layers of the skin and mucosa may form haemangiomata on the cutaneous and mucosal surfaces. On examination of the deeper organs and tissues widespread vascular dilatation and oedema are found.

Clinical Features. The onset may be gradual or acute, affecting a group of people taking the same diet. A period of ill-health with nausea, vomiting and diarrhoea often precedes the onset of the oedema which appears first in the legs and feet and is accompanied by symptoms of cardiac failure. Fever often accompanies the early stage of the illness. In severe cases the pulse is rapid and may be irregular, and signs and symptoms of severe cardiac failure develop. If death occurs it is usually due to heart failure. An erythematous mottling of the skin may follow the oedema, and haemangiomatous tumours up to 1 cm. in diameter may appear in the skin or mucosal surfaces. Bleeding from these after slight trauma is easily controlled by local pressure. Glaucoma is a serious complication.

Diagnosis. During an outbreak the diagnosis is easy from the dietetic history and clinical findings. In contrast to the oedema of beriberi there are no accompanying features of peripheral neuropathy and there is no response to thiamine. Famine oedema attacks those who have been subjected to severe food restriction and who are usually emaciated and hungry.

Treatment. For the affection of the heart, rest in bed is essential and the intake of salt should be restricted. A high protein diet must be given and all contaminated mustard oil excluded. The addition of vitamin B complex to the diet is advisable. Improvement is often slow and convalescence protracted. When ocular tension is increased, surgical treatment is usually required to relieve the tension.

Prevention. Steps should be taken to prevent contamination of mustard crops with the weed *A. mexicana*. A test should be carried out to detect this contaminant in mustard oil.

VOMITING SICKNESS OF JAMAICA
(Ackee Poisoning)

This illness is attributed to the eating of unripe fruit of a common West Indian and South American tree, *Blighia sapida*. The mature fruit is wholesome but unripe fruit is believed to contain hypoglycin, a water-soluble toxin.

Clinical Features. Only children from 2 to 5 years of age who are undernourished are affected. The first symptom is vomiting, and after an interval this is followed by drowsiness, going on to convulsions and coma. In the late stages of the illness there is marked hypoglycaemia which may be due to hypoglycin blocking gluconeogenesis in the liver.

Treatment. If started early, continuous intravenous glucose can bring about recovery. Without treatment the mortality rate is high.

EFFECTS OF LIGHT AND HEAT
Exposure to Strong Sunlight

Sunburn is caused not by the heat of the sun but by ultraviolet light. The skin of those with fair complexions is especially sensitive to strong sunlight. Natural tolerance to the sun can be won by gradual exposure which enables the skin to acquire protective pigmentation.

Clinical Features. Short periods of exposure to unaccustomed strong sun produce only erythema and itchiness of the affected area of skin.

Should, however, the exposure be prolonged, acute pain and oedema with vesicles and bullae soon develop in the affected part. These local changes are accompanied by general malaise, headache and nausea. Severe cases may suffer from prostration and even some cardiovascular failure. When a large area of skin has been damaged, this may interfere seriously with sweating and predispose to heat hyperpyrexia.

Treatment. For mild sunburn no treatment is needed, but for severe cases treatment in bed in a cool room is required with sedatives to relieve the pain. Any features of shock and dehydration must receive the appropriate treatment. Large blisters should be pricked, and calamine lotion containing 0·5 per cent. crystal violet should be applied. Antihistamine drugs given by mouth help to relieve pruritus.

Prophylaxis. Untanned skin should be exposed to strong sunlight only for short graded periods. Some protection is afforded by face powders and creams containing para-aminobenzoic acid which absorbs ultraviolet light.

Solar Keratosis

After prolonged residence in the tropics atrophic patches are liable to develop on exposed parts of the body especially in those with fair skins. The backs of the hands, the neck and the forehead are most commonly affected. These areas may later develop small patches of hyperkeratosis which occasionally progress to the formation of squamous celled carcinomata. This process is seen with maximum severity in albinos in the tropics.

Treatment. The skin should be protected as far as possible from the sunlight by clothing and creams. When the hyperkeratotic areas become troublesome they can be removed by diathermy.

Acclimatisation to Heat

In cool climates heat production in the body is balanced by loss from the surface chiefly by radiation and convection. The hypothalamus controls the superficial circulation and produces vasoconstriction or dilatation as required for the conservation or loss of body heat. When, however, the atmospheric temperature is above that of the body, then evaporation of sweat is all-important in the maintenance of a stable body temperature, assisted to a minor degree by insensible loss through the skin and lungs.

Acclimatisation to heat is an essential preparation for workers exposed to excessive heat in certain industries in cool climates as well as for people who live in the tropics. This can be achieved by undertaking exercise daily under artificially produced or natural hot weather conditions for 10 to 14 days, by the end of which time the body metabolism will have become partially adjusted. As the result of this adjustment an increase in the total volume of circulating fluid compensates the body for the expanded vascular bed, and this is accompanied by a diminished pulse rate and an increased cardiac output. Further, the salt excreted by the kidneys is decreased and in addition the concentration of salt in the sweat is much reduced, mainly as a result of increased activity of the adrenal glands with enhanced production of aldosterone. The sweat glands also become more active, responding more rapidly and efficiently to any increase in body temperature; consequently the rise in body temperature in response to exercise diminishes. With these adjustments the individual is better able to work and remain well under conditions of high atmospheric temperature provided an adequate intake of water and salt is maintained. In contrast, exposure to adverse conditions or the taking of cholinergic drugs may produce cessation of sweating from failure ('fatigue') of the sweat glands.

Prickly Heat

Many Europeans living in the tropics, especially when humidity is high, suffer from prickly heat. Some become acclimatised, while others continue to be troubled by it throughout the hot season. The condition arises from blockage of sweat ducts within the prickle cell layer of the epidermis. As a result of this blockage, sweat escapes into the epidermis and causes severe irritation. The lesions produced consist of numerous minute papules, surrounded by erythema (miliaria rubra) which become vesicular or pustular (miliaria pustulosa). These minute pustules usually contain sterile pus, although scratching may lead to secondary pyogenic infection of them. The lesions of prickly heat are most numerous in parts of the body in close contact with clothing, e.g. around the waist, shoulders or wrists, but they also occur on exposed areas such as the backs of the hands. The lesions are very prickly and irritating and, if extensive, cause great discomfort and may be followed by tropical anhidrotic asthenia. Sweating due to any cause aggravates the symptoms.

Treatment. The principles of treatment are to reduce sweating to a minimum and to overcome the blockage of the sweat ducts. If the patient can be transferred to a cool environment such as an air-conditioned room, the blocked ducts become patent within a week or two. The general measures prescribed below under prophylaxis should be instituted. The skin should be washed gently and the sparing use of a bland soap containing hexochlorophane is helpful. In severe cases, when artificial cooling cannot be maintained, the application of anhydrous lanoline will restore the patency of the sweat ducts.   When irritation is intense relief should be given by the administration of a sedative, such as phenobarbitone, 30 mg. every six hours.

Prophylaxis.   It is important to avoid plugging the orifices of the sweat ducts.   Therefore maceration of the skin by sweat or liquid applications, excessive washing and irritation from clothing (either by friction or a chemical contaminant) must be avoided.   The use of a bland soap containing hexochlorophane is advocated.   Dusting powders should only be lightly applied.   Clothing must be loose fitting, changed frequently and thoroughly rinsed after washing.   Controlled tanning of the skin with sunlight may help acclimatisation.   The diet should be such as does not lead to capillary dilatation and excessive sweating.   Curries, condiments and alcohol should be taken only in moderation, if at all.

Heat Syncope

Heat syncope or fainting is not uncommon in people dressed in unsuitable clothes in a warm atmosphere with poor air circulation, at exercise, on suddenly standing up, after standing still for a considerable time, or even at rest.   Fainting is then due to an expanded vascular bed with an inadequate compensatory increase in blood volume and insufficient cardiac output.   This results in a sudden drop in blood pressure which leads to temporary cerebral anoxia.

Treatment.   The patient is put to rest lying down (the head low and the feet raised) in a cool atmosphere and unnecessary clothing loosened or removed.

Heat Exhaustion

Heat exhaustion is often brought on by a period of great heat or by extra effort under conditions of hot weather, when the patient has not taken enough fluid and salt to balance the increased loss by sweating. The amount of fluid lost as sweat during a working spell under these conditions may be as much as 6 or even 8 litres and even in persons fully acclimatised to heat this may entail a loss of approximately 2 g. sodium chloride per litre of sweat.   Ill-health, especially gastrointestinal disturbances with vomiting and diarrhoea, will increase the risk of heat exhaustion.

Clinical Features.   There are usually warnings which should be recognised.   These include headache, giddiness, loss of appetite, nausea, muscular cramps, especially of the legs and feet, and personality changes— irritability and lack of co-operation.   If the disorder is recognised at this early stage, removal to a cool atmosphere and cool water to drink, with salt as required, will soon restore the patient to normal. If, however, it is not recognised and if treatment is delayed, the results are less satisfactory. In an established case of heat exhaustion the patient is distressed and anxious, with a pale sweating skin, rapid weak pulse and low blood pressure, and often complains of cramps. Although the surface is cool, the rectal temperature may be slightly raised (the 'cold moist man'). Dehydration is usually marked and no chlorides can be found in the high coloured scanty urine, indicating that there is a depletion of both salt and water. When dehydration is limited to loss of extracellular fluid there will be no thirst and consequently a considerable degree of water depletion may exist without producing any symptoms. The importance of water depletion must be stressed. Adequate salt replacement, however, is also essential.

Treatment. In severe cases it is usually not possible to give the required amount of fluid and electrolytes by mouth. Intravenous infusion of saline is therefore needed, the quantity and composition depending on the degree of dehydration and electrolyte deficiency (p. **214**). Useful practical guidance to the requirement of sodium chloride can be obtained by testing the output of chloride in the urine. Initial and maintenance treatment should be carried out in a cool place until convalescence is complete. When heat exhaustion is not recognised and treated, the patient may develop a high temperature and pass into a condition of secondary heat hyperpyrexia (p. 132).

Tropical Anhidrotic Asthenia

The majority of patients with this disorder have suffered from prickly heat. This has left extensive areas of skin, especially on the trunk and limbs, incapable of sweating properly. The condition develops insidiously towards the end of the hot weather, with headache, giddiness, lack of energy, diminished sweating and often marked polyuria, the dilute urine containing chloride. A rise of body temperature is common and may occasionally reach hyperpyrexia. The plasma chlorides are usually only slightly decreased.

Prolonged treatment is needed. The patient must live in a cool climate (for example a change to a hill station) until the skin has recovered and sweating has returned to normal; this may take up to two months.

Heat Hyperpyrexia

Heat hyperpyrexia occurs in those exposed for considerable periods to unusually high atmospheric temperatures, independent of exposure to direct sunlight. Unacclimatised people are more liable to suffer, but a prolonged period of very high temperature may affect even those who are fully acclimatised, including the local inhabitants. The disorder is always associated with cessation of sweating, and then the body temperature may reach 42° to 43° C. (107° to 110° F.) or even higher. Predisposing factors are those which interfere with the production and evaporation of sweat—unsuitable clothing and poor working conditions with little air movement, heavy work in conditions of high temperature and humidity and fever especially when due to malaria, pulmonary or renal disease. Diffuse lesions of the skin, especially if treated with oily preparations and protective coverings, may inhibit sweating and induce heat hyperpyrexia. Individuals with congenital absence of sweat glands are particularly vulnerable. Alcohol and certain drugs like atropine may play a part. Operations, particularly thyroidectomy, may be dangerous. Hyperpyrexia may follow heat exhaustion when the dehydration leads to cessation of sweating.

Pathology. The most important changes are in the central nervous system. There is general congestion of the brain with increased pressure of the cerebrospinal fluid. Microscopic examination may show degeneration of nerve cells, particularly in the hypothalamic region and base of the brain.

Clinical Features. In primary hyperpyrexia the onset is usually dramatic with no warning in a person who appears to be neither dehydrated nor deficient in salt though occasionally the patient may have noticed that perspiration had become much less. He may have retired to rest feeling quite well and be found in coma a few hours later. Loss of consciousness may be preceded by prodromal signs of cerebral irritation. On examination a dry burning skin is found (the 'hot dry man'). When the temperature, which must always be taken rectally, reaches between 41° and 42° C. (105° and 107° F.) unconsciousness supervenes and without energetic treatment the mortality rate can be 50 per cent. Heat hyperpyrexia may be complicated by peripheral circulatory failure or acute renal or hepatic failure. Haemorrhages are a frequent feature. After death the temperature may continue to rise.

In cases of secondary hyperpyrexia the early symptoms are those of heat exhaustion or tropical anhidrotic asthenia. If the patient is not treated, the temperature continues to rise and the state of hyperpyrexia supervenes.

Diagnosis. Heat hyperpyrexia is likely during any prolonged period of unusually hot atmospheric conditions. Any patient with an unduly high temperature and dry skin should be treated as such a case, care being taken to exclude other diseases, especially *P. falciparum* malaria by a careful blood examination. A neutrophil leucocytosis is present. Lumbar puncture will exclude meningitis and at the same time will relieve the increased cerebrospinal fluid pressure so frequent in heat hyperpyrexia.

Treatment. The aim is to reduce the temperature as quickly as possible in order to prevent permanent damage to vital structures. This is done by loosely wrapping the patient in a cool wet sheet and promoting evaporation by fanning. Concurrently parenteral antimalarial therapy (p. **1120)** should be given if malaria is a possibility. As the temperature falls, provided that the brain has not been irreparably damaged, consciousness returns. Cooling should be stopped when the rectal temperature has fallen to around 39° C. (102° F.), otherwise the temperature, which goes on falling, may reach excessively low levels. As anoxia is frequently present oxygen should be given. Chlorpromazine should be administered and an adequate airway maintained. When return to consciousness is delayed, lumbar puncture and withdrawal of excess fluid may help. In the presence of circulatory failure intravenous hydrocortisone may be life saving. For the treatment of acute renal or hepatic failure see pages **725** and **645**. During convalescence control of body temperature will remain unstable.

When hyperpyrexia is secondary to heat exhaustion, dehydration is usually severe. Therefore, in addition to reducing the high temperature, adequate water and salt replacement is essential.

Depending on the duration and degree of hyperpyrexia, the patient may recover completely, be left with residual brain damage or fail to respond to treatment.

Prevention of Ill-effects of Heat

Careful selection should be made of those required to work under hot atmospheric conditions. General physical fitness and mental stability are important; people in the younger age group are, as a rule, more suitable for such employment. Fever, gastrointestinal upsets, alcoholic excess and lack of sleep all predispose to ill-effects of heat. It is highly important that the skin should be healthy and that sweating should be normal.

When the atmospheric temperature is very high, leading to excessive sweating, even the fully acclimatised require to take extra fluid and salt. A daily intake of up to as much as 15 litres of cool drinking water and 30 g. of sodium chloride per person may be needed to prevent water and salt depletion. Advice and encouragement is usually required if such large amounts of fluid are to be taken. The extra salt is usually taken with food and in the drinking water, but it can, when necessary, be supplied in enteric coated tablets. A total of 30 g. of sodium chloride is supplied by adding 3 flat teaspoonfuls of salt or 18 enteric coated tablets, each containing 650 mg. of salt, to the normal daily intake of fluid and food.

In addition, everything possible should be done to improve working conditions by arranging for a free circulation of air and for a reduction of high temperature and excessive atmospheric humidity by means of air-conditioning. Clothing should be light and loose fitting. Hard or prolonged manual work should not be undertaken when atmospheric conditions are exceptionally unfavourable. Off-duty living conditions should be made as cool and comfortable as possible.

TROPICAL SPRUE

Sprue is the name which the Dutch in Java gave to a tropical disease in which the presenting features are sore mouth, fatty diarrhoea and associated secondary manifestations of subnutrition and malnutrition. The cause is unknown.

Although delayed and defective absorption of fat is the abnormality most easily recognised, the absorption of water, sodium chloride, glucose, vitamins and minerals is also impaired (see below). The absorption of amino acids is less affected and the excretion of pancreatic enzymes is normal.

Aetiology. The disease is widespread in the tropics, especially in some parts of Asia including Ceylon, Southern India, Malaysia, Indonesia, Hong Kong and China. It also occurs in the Middle East, in certain of the Caribbean Islands and in South America but is extremely rare, if it occurs at all, in tropical Africa. It occurs frequently in Europeans and in Indians; it is also seen in Malays and Caribbeans of Spanish descent, but is rare in Chinese. It has also been reported in Puerto Rico, but whether these patients had sprue or nutritional megaloblastic anaemia is not clear (see below). In so far as epidemiology is concerned sprue may be considered under four headings.

GROUP 1. In the century before the Second World War tropical sprue as it occurred in Java, Hong Kong, Singapore and Colombo was a disease which appeared to be largely confined to Europeans, usually of middle age, most of whom had lived many years in the tropics and who were financially well off compared to the local inhabitants because of their professional and business incomes. The disease occurred sporadically and usually developed insidiously and was notable for remissions and relapses, often for no obvious reason. A return to temperate climates usually caused a remission but relapses occurred sometimes after many years' absence from the tropics. Epidemics of sprue were not reported but the occurrence of sprue in successive residents in a particular house (sprue houses) suggested an infective cause.

There is no doubt that the incidence of tropical sprue in Europeans resident in endemic areas in Asia such as Colombo and Singapore is much less than formerly. During this period of falling incidence there has been a great increase in the number of refrigerators in shops, hotels and private houses, and also as large industrial cold storage plants. Whether this reduced incidence of sprue is due to improved hygiene consequent upon the increased use of refrigeration or whether the quality of foods, both imported and home grown, has been beneficially influenced is a matter of conjecture. The primary cause of this pre-war type of sprue has never been elucidated and no specific agent, toxic, infective or nutritional, has been found.

GROUP 2. Sprue in Puerto Rico is a disease which has been known for a long time; it affected the poorest inhabitants, whose diet was grossly defective in many respects. The megaloblastic anaemia which was present in many cases was shown by Spies many years ago to respond dramatically to folic acid, which had recently been synthesised, with corresponding beneficial effects on the gastrointestinal and other clinical features. Sprue in Puerto Rico was believed by many to be a primary nutritional deficiency disease due mainly to folic acid deficiency. More recently American military personnel in Puerto Rico have developed tropical sprue in spite of consuming an excellent diet. The question therefore arises whether sprue in American soldiers in Puerto Rico is the same disease as occurred in the grossly malnourished poor inhabitants.

GROUP 3. During the Second World War when hundreds of thousands of troops went to S.E. Asia sprue was reported to have occurred in epidemics both in British and Indian soldiers, some of whom had only been in the area for days or weeks. They had previously been eating excellent Army rations and were much younger in age than those classical cases of sprue in group 1. The onset was often sudden in contrast to the insidious onset of group 1.

GROUP 4. Baker described a large epidemic of sprue in Indians in 1961-62 in Vellore, Southern India. This epidemic has subsided but the disease is still endemic in that area. The cases had the classical features of sprue. Despite the obvious suggestion that an epidemic of this size must have an infective basis, no specific organisms were found, but the possibility remains that it was due to some unidentified virus. Since the Indian population in South India has been partaking of a notoriously poor diet for a long time and since no change in the diet occurred during the epidemic or after it had ceased, the view that this form of sprue was primarily due to dietary deficiency received no support.

The view that tropical sprue is a specific nutritional disease primarily due to dietary deficiency of folic acid cannot be sustained for several reasons.

Thus it has been fully substantiated that severe nutritional megaloblastic anaemia due to folic acid deficiency is of common occurrence in tropical Africa where tropical sprue is virtually unknown. Likewise the megaloblastic anaemia of pregnant women which is a common disorder in many parts of the world is primarily due to folic acid deficiency but fatty diarrhoea is not a feature. Hence it must be concluded that the clinical features of sprue are primarily the result of malabsorption due to some as yet unknown cause or causes.

This primary defect in absorption may be increased by any associated bacterial gastrointestinal infection or change in the pattern of the bacterial flora of the small intestine. An attack of sprue frequently follows upon bacillary dysentery or other gastrointestinal infections, but the aetiological association with these diseases has not survived statistical analysis.

Once deficiency of folic acid has occurred, a vicious circle may be commenced as folic acid is required in large amounts by the intestinal cells if the effete cells of the small intestine are to be rapidly replaced by new cells. In other words folic acid deficiency may well be an important factor in maintaining or increasing intestinal malabsorption.

It is difficult to understand why the administration of antibiotics may improve the intestinal features of sprue either when given alone or as a supplement to folic acid therapy, since no specific organisms which could be killed by the antibiotic have been incriminated as the cause of sprue. Perhaps the effect is similar to that produced in the blind loop syndrome (p. 573) in which organisms divert vitamin B_{12} to their own use and thus make the patient deficient in this vitamin. If sprue is due to a virus it seems unlikely that it would be killed by any antibiotic at present available.

The discovery that wheat-gluten is the agent responsible for coeliac disease (gluten enteropathy) indicates the possibility that some constitutional inability to deal with certain nutrients may be important. Thus it has been suggested that the explanation of the geographical location of tropical sprue in Ceylon, India, Indonesia and China and its absence in Africa, may be correlated with the foods eaten, including the type of fat used for cooking, in these regions.

Patients with tropical sprue are not sensitive to wheat-gluten and its withdrawal from the diet produces no clinical benefit.

The clinical and biochemical abnormalities and the radiological and histological changes in the small intestine in sprue are not specific for that disease, since comparable findings are present in other malabsorptive disorders such as coeliac disease (gluten enteropathy) and non-tropical sprue (idiopathic steatorrhoea).

From what has been said it may be concluded (1) that the cause of tropical sprue is not known and (2) that the condition may be a clinical syndrome rather than a disease entity.

Pathology. The pathological changes closely resemble those of wheat-gluten sensitivity, although they tend to be less advanced. The jejunal villi are blunted or rarely absent and there may be a subepithelial cellular infiltration with plasma cells and lymphocytes. This appearance, called partial villous atrophy, is a non-specific change and may be found in other diseases of the small intestine with steatorrhoea. The abnormality appears to be confined to the jejunum in early sprue but later also affects the ileum.

The stores of vitamin B_{12} in the body are much greater than those of folate, probably enough for two to three years. As this vitamin is absorbed from the lower ileum, which is much less affected in sprue than the jejunum, a deficiency of vitamin B_{12} takes longer to develop and is encountered only in sprue of long duration. A macrocytic anaemia is common in sprue and in many cases megaloblastic change is present in the bone marrow. In the earlier stages of the disease this appears to be due to folate deficiency alone. When malabsorption has continued for weeks or months deficiencies of other vitamins such as A, D and K and riboflavin may result. The clinical and biochemical signs of depletion of water and minerals, including especially iron and calcium but also sodium, potassium and magnesium, may also be present.

Clinical Features. The condition can present in any grade of clinical severity. Although the onset may be acute and occur within a few weeks of arrival in the tropics, it is more often insidious with increasing lassitude, mental apathy and depression, loss of weight, anorexia, flatulence and dyspepsia. Remissions and relapses which occur for no obvious cause are a characteristic feature. Initially or after some weeks a watery explosive diarrhoea occurs which in some cases appears to have been precipitated by a gastrointestinal infection or by dietary or alcoholic indiscretion. Later, up to 10 pale loose foul smelling stools may be passed daily, especially in the morning or during the night. Defaecation is urgent, follows meals and the stool is bulky, frothy, floats in the lavatory pan and is difficult to flush away. Vomiting may occur with nausea, abdominal distension and borborygmi. After some time the tongue becomes sore, first at the tip and edges, the discomfort being increased by smoking or taking hot spicy food and curries; it becomes fiery red in colour and painful. Later the whole mouth and throat feel sore and there may be difficulty in swallowing. Nocturnal urinary frequency and in women amenorrhoea have been noted.

In the untreated chronic disease there is much loss of weight, the tongue is clean and shiny from atrophy of the filiform papillae and fissures may develop. ·Abdominal distension, pallor and generalised pigmentation appear. The skin becomes coarse and dry (follicular keratosis) possibly due to deficiency of vitamin A (p. **149**). Fever is uncommon unless associated with severe megaloblastic anaemia or with superadded infection, often of the urinary tract. Continued malabsorption of vitamins of the B complex leads to glossitis, cheilosis and angular stomatitis (p. **191**) and rarely lack of absorbed vitamin K causes a tendency to bleed into the skin or from the mucous membranes (p. **167**). Bleeding haemorrhoids may be a feature and complicate the appearance of the stools. Loss of fluids and electrolytes may lead to severe dehydration, muscular weakness and cramps, and lack of vitamin D and calcium to osteomalacia and tetany. Oedema of the extremities may be a feature of the chronic disease. Peripheral neuropathy is very rare.

Diagnosis. The clinical features and the history of residence in an area noted for tropical sprue will suggest the correct diagnosis if care is taken to recognise the early and the mild cases as well as the late presentations. Evidence of malabsorption is obtained by estimation of the faecal fat (on an ordinary ward diet not more than 6 g. of fat is passed daily by the normal person, p. **576**), by the flat glucose tolerance curve (p. **795**) and by the abnormal d-xylose tolerance test (p. **576**). After a 25 g. loading oral dose the normal person excretes 25 per cent. in the urine within five hours. This is also the case in patients with pancreatic steatorrhoea. In contrast, in sprue and wheat-gluten induced enteropathy the percentage excreted is reduced. If the 25 g. dose causes nausea or vomiting a 5 g. loading dose may be used instead.

The anaemia, when present, is usually macrocytic and the bone marrow megaloblastic, but it may also be hypochromic from defective absorption of iron, in which case a dimorphic anaemia is produced (pp. **846**, **848**). Although temporary achlorhydria is not uncommon in sprue it is not usually histamine fast. If free acid is present in the gastric juice after the injection of histamine, pernicious anaemia can be excluded.

Intestinal anatomy is assessed by barium X-ray examination (p. **574**) using non-flocculable barium, and by intestinal biopsy (p. **575**). The histological appearance is that of villous atrophy and neither this nor the radiological signs are specific for tropical sprue but merely indicate that a malabsorption syndrome is present.

Differential diagnosis is from other forms of steatorrhoea such as chronic pancreatitis, wheat-gluten enteropathy (coeliac disease), idiopathic steatorrhoea (non-tropical sprue), regional ileitis and tuberculous enteritis. Lymphoma of the small intestine, pernicious anaemia, gastric carcinoma and Addison's disease may also have to be considered. Malabsorption may also result from heavy infections of the intestine with *Giardia intestin-*

alis or *Strongyloides stercoralis*. Intestinal hurry as part of an allergic response in the early stages of ancylostomiasis may suggest the onset of sprue (p. 81). Early symptoms of sprue may erroneously be attributed to amoebiasis or a neurosis.

Treatment. Complete rest in bed is required initially for the severely affected patient. If diarrhoea is severe a preparation of codeine may be required temporarily. In addition dehydration must be corrected and supplements of potassium may be required. For the patient with disease of recent and acute onset 10 mg. of folic acid is given intramuscularly daily for three days. In addition 5 mg. is given orally twice daily for at least one month after all symptoms have disappeared. This normally produces a dramatic clinical response with rapid improvement in glossitis, stomatitis, steatorrhoea and other clinical features. If the bone marrow is megaloblastic there is a brisk haematological response with reticulocytosis and reversion to normoblastic bone marrow. Serial jejunal biopsies have shown that in recent cases the jejunal mucosa soon returns to normal following folic acid therapy. Such a patient can continue to live in the tropics and remain well. It has not yet been established whether a small dose of folic acid should be given daily to patients remaining in the tropics to prevent a relapse or to administer folic acid only if a relapse occurs.

If untreated sprue has been present for more than six months steatorrhoea will persist in about a quarter of the patients for a variable period despite treatment with folic acid, but this will usually respond to a course of antibiotics. For this purpose 1 g. tetracycline daily for 7-14 days should be given. If there is no response, 2 g. chloramphenicol daily for five days should be tried.

Some patients suffering from long continued chronic sprue may not respond to folic acid because of severe deficiency of vitamin B_{12}. These patients should be given intramuscular injections of hydroxocobalamin, 1000 micrograms twice in one week, followed by a dose of 250 micrograms once a fortnight for six weeks in addition to folic acid. By this means the anaemia is corrected and the danger of developing subacute combined degeneration of the spinal cord is avoided.

If hypochromic anaemia due to iron deficiency is present, ferrous sulphate must be given. In severe cases a multivitamin preparation containing thiamine, 10 mg., riboflavin, 5 mg. and nicotinamide, 50 mg. twice daily should be prescribed for a few weeks. In addition phytomenadione (Vitamin K_1) (p. **167**) will be required if there is a tendency to bleed. Tetany necessitates the giving of calcium parenterally and vitamin D by mouth.

Complicated diets are no longer required but the diet initially should be bland and appetising, limited in fat and carbohydrate and high in protein. Because of their high content of folic acid and other vitamins the importance of liver, meat and green vegetables in the diet must be stressed after recovery. Folic acid supplements should always be given to women who have had sprue should they become pregnant.

FREDERICK J. WRIGHT.
JAMES P. BAIRD.

Anaemia in the Tropics

In many tropical countries anaemia of severe degree is prevalent. This is explained largely by the high frequency of protozoal, helminthic and bacterial infections and the prevalence of malnutrition in the tropics. It cannot be emphasised too strongly that the aetiology of anaemia in the tropics shows great variation from country to country and area to area, and effective management can only follow the clear appreciation of local patterns of disease, nutrition and social custom. It is not the purpose of this chapter to describe those causes of anaemia also seen in temperate climates. These are covered adequately in the section dealing with disorders of the blood in *The Principles and Practice of Medicine* (pp. **828** to **891**). The reader is referred to the chapter dealing with nutritional diseases for information regarding nutritional deficiency as a cause of anaemia (pp. **123** to **212**).

IRON DEFICIENCY ANAEMIA

ANCYLOSTOMIASIS. This is a major cause of iron deficiency anaemia. Each worm ingests between 0·03 and 0·15 ml. of blood per day; hence the loss of blood in a heavy infection (over 1,000 worms) is large, and anaemia develops rapidly after the iron stores are exhausted. Folic acid deficiency may complicate the anaemia if the dietary intake is inadequate for the demands of increased red cell formation. Where the blood loss is severe protein deficiency may also appear. However, this last complication is unlikely to occur in the face of reasonable nutrition and adequate liver function. If the anaemia is treated with iron it rapidly improves, but will return when iron therapy is stopped, unless deworming is undertaken. It follows that deworming is essential in treating the anaemia (pp. 80 to 83).

Because of the mode of infection, ancylostomiasis predominantly affects the agricultural communities. Hookworm infection sufficient to cause anaemia does not usually occur in children under 2 years of age.

In addition all the usual features of iron deficiency anaemia, namely angular stomatitis, glossitis and koilonychia may be seen and kwashiorkor may complicate the picture (pp. **191, 837** and **130**).

The aetiology, prevention and treatment of ancylostomiasis is described on pages 80 to 83.

MEGALOBLASTIC ANAEMIA

Although Addisonian pernicious anaemia (p. **844**) occurs in all races, it is relatively uncommon in tropical countries, where megaloblastic anaemia is much more frequently due to nutritional deficiency of folic acid or vitamin B_{12}. The requirements of both these substances are increased during growth, pregnancy, infections (including malaria) and when there is increased red cell formation as in haemolytic anaemia. Generally, in this respect the available body store of folic acid is more vulnerable to depletion than that of vitamin B_{12}, hence most instances of megaloblastic anaemia in the tropics are due to folic acid deficiency. Where animal protein is nearly or completely absent from the diet, vitamin B_{12} deficiency may occur.

Diagnosis. There are no particular clinical features indicative of megaloblastic anaemia, but persistent diarrhoea and vomiting in infants with resultant failure to thrive is often corrected only when folic acid is given. Megaloblastic anaemia should always be suspected when anaemia complicates malnutrition or under-nutrition, or persists in spite of adequate treatment of an acute infection in infants. Anaemia in pregnancy in the tropics is a result of a combination of many causes, but folic acid deficiency is usually a major factor and may occur as early as the twentieth week of gestation.

The finding of a neurological disorder, particularly mental apathy and peripheral neuritis, and the presence of increased pigmentation of the palmar skin should suggest vitamin B_{12} deficiency.

Iron deficiency frequently co-exists with megaloblastic anaemia. Thus the typical blood appearances of macrocytic red cells well filled with haemoglobin may be modified by the presence of hypochromic and microcytic forms (dimorphic anaemia, p. **846**). The occurrence of hypersegmentation of the nuclei of the polymorph leucocytes is unfortunately not diagnostic of megaloblastic change, as it may occur in iron deficiency states, but its presence should raise strong suspicions. Confirmation should be obtained, whenever possible, by the examination of a bone marrow aspirate.

If vitamin B_{12} deficiency is suspected, the presence of free hydrochloric acid in the gastric aspirate after administering pentagastrin will exclude Addisonian pernicious anaemia (p. **844**).

Treatment. Most cases will respond completely to folic acid (5 to 15 mg./day) by mouth. If vitamin B_{12} deficiency is considered likely it is wise to give hydroxocobalamin by intramuscular injection (250 micrograms each week) until an adequate dietary intake is assured. Iron should also be given orally in the usual doses (p. **840**). In the majority of cases continued treatment is unnecessary, but in pregnancy folic acid should be given until after delivery. If achlorhydria has been demonstrated and Addisonian pernicious anaemia is presumed or confirmed, it is necessary to continue treatment with hydroxocobalamin throughout life. In remote areas or in other circumstances which make regular injections impossible, a daily oral dose of 300 micrograms of cyanocobalamin is a satisfactory, although probably inferior method of vitamin B_{12} administration.

Prevention. Because of the frequency of deficiency it is wise to add folic acid (5 mg. daily) to the treatment of all infants with kwashiorkor or other forms of malnutrition, with infections or with haemolytic anaemia. Similarly 350 micrograms folic acid and 100 mg. of elemental iron should be given daily from as early as possible throughout pregnancy.

HAEMOLYTIC ANAEMIA

The various types of haemolytic anaemia which occur in temperate climates are also encountered in tropical countries. In addition haemolytic anaemia in the tropics is frequently due to malaria or other infections. Two types of genetic abnormality resulting in haemolytic anaemia are also particularly common and are therefore dealt with in detail here; they are the deficiency of the enzyme glucose-6-phosphate dehydrogenase and the haemoglobinopathies.

MALARIA. An attack of malarial fever, especially when due to *Plasmodium falciparum*, is always accompanied by haemolysis, and in a severe or prolonged attack very considerable anaemia may ensue. The destruction of red cells in malaria is always in excess of that caused by parasitised cells. The reason for this is ill-understood although it is most likely to be due to an immune mechanism. Generally, the degree of the anaemia is related to the severity of the parasitaemia. During an acute attack of malaria the reticulocyte count may be low but as the patient recovers a brisk outpouring of young red cells occurs. This recuperative response may be embarrassed by deficiency states, especially of folic acid and iron, or by other infections. Where these occur anaemia will be more severe and prolonged.

A district can be classified according to the intensity of malaria in it, as hypoendemic, mesoendemic, hyperendemic or holoendemic (p. **1118**). In hyperendemic or holoendemic zones little anaemia is produced in the indigenous peoples over the age of 5 to 7 years, because of the development of a high degree of tolerance to the parasites ('premunity'). This tolerance is known to be prejudiced by the prolonged use of suppressive drugs or residence in malaria free areas, in pregnancy, following splenectomy and in diseases of the reticulo-endothelial system such as lymphoma. Under these circumstances anaemia may be seen in those previously immune. Anaemia occurs mostly in the non-immune or weakly immune, such as visitors, young children and adults living in areas of malarial hypoendemicity or mesoendemicity. In such patients splenomegaly may be a prominent feature. It follows from what has been said that in areas of low endemicity treatment of malarial anaemia in the population is likely to be of only transient benefit unless accompanied by eradication of the malaria. On the other hand, in areas of high endemicity, unless eradication can effectively eliminate the infection, there is the risk of creating an area of low endemicity with the subsequent increase in malarial anaemia that would follow the inevitable drop in individual immunity.

BLACKWATER FEVER, OROYA FEVER, SNAKE VENOM. Anaemia resulting from haemolysis occurs in blackwater fever (a complication of neglected falciparum malaria, p. **1118**), in acute bartonellosis (Oroya fever, p. 17) and as a result of the venom of certain snakes (p. 111).

Glucose-6-phosphate Dehydrogenase Deficiency

Haemolytic anaemia following the ingestion of 8-aminoquinoline drugs used against malaria was observed in about 10 per cent. of American Negro troops in Korea. This was shown to be due to a deficiency in the red cells of the enzyme glucose-6-phosphate dehydrogenase. As a result of this lack of enzyme, the red cells fail to keep their glutathione in the reduced state and as a consequence are unable to maintain their integrity when appropriately challenged. It is now known that the deficiency is inherited as a sex-linked recessive and has a high frequency among Negroes. In West and East Africa about 20 per cent. of males are affected, and about 4 per cent. of females are homozygous for the abnormal gene and are therefore also deficient. Many drugs in common clinical use, e.g. 8-aminoquinolines and other antimalarials, sulphonamides, sulphones, acetylsalicylic acid, phenacetin, para-amino-salicylic acid, chloramphenicol and even vitamin K, are capable of precipitating haemolysis in individuals with this defect. Infections may also have this effect.

The discovery that favism (haemolytic anaemia resulting from the ingestion of the broad bean, *Vicia faba*) was due to deficiency of glucose-6-phosphate dehydrogenase, indicated that this enzyme deficiency occurred also in some inhabitants of the Mediterranean littoral. There are both electrophoretic and quantitative differences in activity between the enzyme in Negro and Caucasian deficient patients. In Negroes the activity of the enzyme is about 15 per cent. of that in non-deficient subjects whereas in Caucasians it is often less than 1 per cent. Thus the clinical effects are greater in the Caucasian type of deficiency. Recently some hitherto unexplained cases of haemolytic disease of the newborn have also been attributed to the same defect. Yet other types of glucose-6-phosphate dehydrogenase biochemically different from the above may be associated with congenital nonspherocytic haemolytic disease and have been found in persons of pure British ancestry. In these cases it is important to realise that splenectomy is valueless. Persons with this enzyme deficiency normally enjoy good health, but are liable to haemolysis if any of the precipitating drugs or foods are injected or ingested. The anaemia is rapid in onset, usually becoming clinically obvious about 3 to 10 days after exposure to the precipitating agent. There is evidence that the degree of haemolysis may be related to the dose of the agent. It may be sufficiently severe to cause haemoglobinuria as well as the other classical signs of haemolysis, namely hyperbilirubinaemia of the unconjugated type, raised reticulocyte count, nucleated red cells in the peripheral blood, absent haptoglobins and methaemalbuminaemia. In the Negro-type of deficiency only cells of a certain age and over are involved, so that the haemolysis is to some extent self-limiting, even when the offending drug is continued. Young red cells do have some glucose-6-phosphate dehydrogenase activity, and remain viable until their enzyme complement decays when they become susceptible to haemolysis. Since in the Caucasian variety the enzyme activity of young cells is negligible the destruction is more disastrous. Anuria is an infrequent but serious complication. The diagnosis can be confirmed by estimating the enzyme activity of the red cells. If anaemia is severe, tranfusion of red cells with normal enzyme activity is necessary. More usually recovery occurs rapidly once the offending agent is withdrawn or reduced in dose. As stated above, females may be homozygous for the gene resulting in glucose-6-phosphate dehydrogenase deficiency, they may be homozygous for the allelomorphic normal gene or they may be heterozygous. Heterozygotes show enzyme level varying from normal to levels as low as are found in deficient subjects. Those with very low levels suffer from haemolysis when provoked in the same way as deficient males and can be detected by the simple screening tests. Heterozygotes with higher amounts of the enzyme can only be detected by the actual assay methods and do not generally suffer from haemolysis even when provoked.

The survival of a harmful gene in high frequency can only be due to it conferring an advantage to the heterozygote. As in the case of the sickling gene (p. 147) glucose-6-phosphate dehydrogenase deficiency is common only in areas of the world where falciparum malaria was, at least until recently, endemic. But direct evidence that deficiency of this enzyme protects against death from malaria is not nearly so convincing as in the case of sickling. Whereas death from cerebral malaria is exceptionally rare in heterozygotes for sickle-cell haemoglobin, it has been reported in children with glucose-6-phosphate dehydrogenase deficiency but not as frequently as in normal children in the same area.

THE HAEMOGLOBINOPATHIES

Sickle-cell Anaemia

Sickle-cell anaemia has been recognised amongst Negroes and to a lesser extent amongst some inhabitants of the Mediterranean littoral since the beginning of the century. It is only comparatively recently, however, that it was found to be due to the possession of the abnormal haemoglobin designated haemoglobin S.

It is now known that abnormal haemoglobins result from amino acid substitutions in their polypeptide chains. These in turn reflect mutations in the structural genes controlling the production of these chains. There are four such structural gene loci in humans, all on autosomal chromosomes and therefore paired. They are designated alpha (α), gamma (γ), beta (β) and delta (δ) and are responsible for the production of the three main haemoglobins seen during extra-uterine life, namely haemoglobins F, A and A_2. Each of these haemoglobins contains in common two α chains, and their differences reflect the possession of two γ chains in the case of haemoglobin F, two β chains in haemoglobin A and two δ chains in haemoglobin A_2. Thus, the globin fraction of these three types of haemoglobin may be written $\alpha_2\gamma_2$, $\alpha_2\beta_2$ and $\alpha_2\delta_2$ respectively. Each chain in the globin fraction carries one haem moiety in its folds.

Alpha chains possess 141 amino acids in sequence, and γ, β and δ chains 146. Amino acid substitutions may occur at any point along these chains. Each chain has an 'N' and a 'C' terminal and the polypeptide chains are numbered starting from the 'N' terminal. More than one kind of amino acid substitution can occur at one point. For example the substitution of valine for glutamic acid at the N_6 position of the β chain produces haemoglobin S, whereas if the substitution is lysine haemoglobin C results. The beta chains of haemoglobin A are designated βA and those of haemoglobin S and C, βS and βC respectively. Sickle cell haemoglobin should be written $\alpha_2 A \beta_2 S$. However, it is convenient and practical when dealing with the common abnormal haemoglobins to represent them simply by the capital letter A, S, C and E and so on. As there are now well over 100 haemoglobin variants known, the letters of the alphabet do not suffice and for some years new variants have been given names, often of the towns or districts in which they were discovered. Sickle-cell haemoglobin is the most important, but haemoglobins C, D$_{PUNJAB}$ and E are also important in the areas of the world where they occur, particularly when inherited together with haemoglobin S or with β-thalassaemia.

An individual's haemoglobin is inherited from both parents. Thus, a normal adult can be represented as having the haemoglobin phenotype AA. Sickle-cell trait is represented by AS and sickle-cell anaemia, or homozygous haemoglobin S disease, by SS. The inheritance can be graphically shown thus:

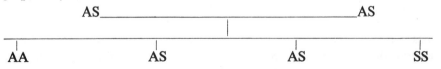

AS_____AS

AA   AS   AS   SS

There is a high incidence of persons with sickle-cell haemoglobin in equatorial Africa; in many countries, e.g. Nigeria and Uganda over 20 per cent. of adults have the trait (i.e. Hb.AS). About 9 per cent. of American and West Indian Negroes have the trait and it is also found in inhabitants of some areas of North Africa, Greece, Southern Italy, the Middle East and Southern India. As most of the homozygotes die before reaching puberty it is surprising that the genetic abnormality has persisted. This has now been explained by the concept of balanced polymorphism. By this is meant that the heterozygote (AS) must have a better chance of surviving than the normal homozygote (AA) to compensate for the increased death rate of the abnormal homozygotes (SS). It is now known that the heterozygote is unlikely to die from falciparum malaria. This explains the high frequency of survival of the haemoglobin S gene in those areas of the world where falciparum malaria was, until recently, endemic.

Clinical Features. An understanding of the pathology and symptomatology of sickle-cell anaemia must be based on a knowledge of the properties of the abnormal haemoglobin. When haemoglobin S is deoxygenated the molecules of haemoglobin polymerise to form pseudo-crystalline structures known as 'tactoids'. As these form they distort the red cell membrane and produce the characteristic sickle shape of the cells. The polymerisation is reversible when re-oxygenation occurs. The greater the concentration of sickle-cell haemoglobin in the individual cell, the more easily are 'tactoids' formed.

In homozygous S disease (sickle-cell anaemia) most of the red cells contain haemoglobin S and little else and are very prone to 'sickle' even *in vivo* under normal conditions. This happens particularly in those parts of the micro-vasculature where, for one reason or another, flow is sluggish. Sickled cells traverse capillaries poorly and tend to block the flow thus increasing the sickling of other cells and causing cessation of flow. Thrombosis may follow and an area of tissue infarction results associated with severe pain, swelling and tenderness (pain crisis).

Sickled cells are phagocytosed in large numbers by the reticulo-endothelial system. This is reflected in hepatosplenomegaly which may be marked early in life. Repeated episodes of splenic infarction however, reduce the size of the organ and if the patient survives to adult life the spleen may be impalpable. As a result of the haemolysis the patient is usually jaundiced and this is further increased by the pathological changes in the liver. Occasionally, although surprisingly rarely, pigment gall-stones are formed.

There is a severe haemolytic disorder with a reduction in mean red cell life span from 120 days to as little as 20 days and during crisis even less. The increased haemolysis is continuous and the haemoglobin level seldom rises above 10 g./100 ml. Crises occur in which sequestration and destruction of the red cells is increased. During these periods the patient feels ill and feverish, becomes more jaundiced and the haemoglobin drops rapidly. The liver and spleen enlarge further. Such 'haemolytic crises' do not necessarily coincide with 'pain crises'. Aplastic crises similar to those seen in other chronic haemolytic disorders have also been reported.

The haemolytic anaemia developing in the first few months of life causes considerable marrow hyperplasia, expanding the marrow cavity and producing the bossed appearance of the skull, the protuberant teeth and prominent cheek bones. Radiological examination of the skull shows the 'hair on end' appearance of the vault of the skull. The life-long haemolytic disease and anaemia which averages about 8 g./100 ml. is associated with erythroid hyperplasia and increased demands for folic acid. Megaloblastic change is a common complication in the under-nourished. Where folate deficiency has been long standing growth may be retarded, puberty delayed and the appearance mistaken for pituitary deficiency. Iron deficiency is not common and a large amount of haemosiderin is usually seen in liver, spleen and bone marrow. Chronic cardiomegaly is also common and is attributed to the chronic severe anaemia.

At birth the baby destined to have sickle cell anaemia has no symptoms or signs of the disease. The majority of the red cells carry haemoglobin F. As the switch over to cells carrying the 'adult' type of haemoglobin occurs symptoms and signs appear; anaemia, jaundice and pain crises, the last classically in the fingers and toes which show large fusiform swellings (dactylitis). The metacarpal and metatarsal bones may also be involved. The late results seen in older children are obvious shortening of one or more digits.

During infancy and childhood frequent attacks of painful swellings of the long bones and vertebrae may occur, due to infarction. These are characteristically sudden in onset and often accompanied by increased jaundice. The pain is of such severity as to confine the child to bed and, as fever is an invariable accompaniment, the episode may be mistaken for rheumatic fever. In any one episode more than one bone may be affected. The attacks last 3 to 20 days and usually subside gradually. There is often a fall in the haemoglobin level and this may be sufficiently severe to require blood transfusion. The main complication to be feared is osteomyelitis which is usually due to the *Salmonella* group of organisms. The after effects of repeated infarction of bones can be demonstrated in radiographs of the diaphyseal areas. As the child grows older the frequency of 'bone-pain' crises becomes less, but periodic attacks are the rule throughout life. In older children and in adults superficial ulcers on the medial aspect of the leg, just above the ankle, are common and extremely slow to heal.

Reduced oxygen tension in the pulmonary circulation, due to respiratory tract infection or vascular occlusion with bone marrow emboli, leads to very rapid onset of severe dyspnoea, pulmonary hypertension and massive sequestration of sickled cells in the lungs. These pulmonary crises may be rapidly fatal. If recovery occurs pulmonary fibrosis and cor pulmonale are common sequelae.

If intravascular sickling occurs in the mesenteric vessels, the clinical features of sudden abdominal pain, vomiting, absent bowel sounds, board-like rigidity and fever closely simulate those of peritonitis or other abdominal emergency. Frequent diagnostic mistakes have been made and have led to death as a result of an unnecessary laparotomy.

Thromboses in intracranial vessels will cause cerebral infarction. Since these intracranial thromboses are usually venous, recovery is the rule, but focal epilepsy may be a late sequel. Another not infrequent complication is painless haematuria, due to infarction of the renal papillae.

Diagnosis. The diagnosis should always be suspected in a patient who has had symptoms of anaemia since infancy and who belongs to a race which may be affected with the sickle-cell trait. Enquiry will often reveal a history of episodes of bone pain. Microscopic examination of a stained blood film from a patient with sickle-cell anaemia will show some sickle-shaped red cells but these will not be seen in the blood film from a person who has only the sickle-cell trait. The presence of haemoglobin S can be confirmed by the demonstration that the red cells will sickle within 20 minutes when mixed on a glass slide with a freshly prepared 2 per cent. solution of sodium metabisulphite and covered with a coverslip. Alternatively a small drop of blood diluted in saline may be incubated under a sealed coverslip overnight when sickling will occur. A positive result will occur in the trait and in haemoglobin SC disease as well as in sickle-cell anaemia.

When suspected, the diagnosis should always be confirmed by electro-phoretic analysis of the haemoglobin and, if necessary, by a family study to demonstrate the inheritance. In this way true sickle-cell anaemia can be differentiated from other diseases in which haemoglobin S is combined with thalassaemia or some other abnormal haemoglobin such as C or D.

Treatment. There is no method of changing the genetic make-up of an individual and therefore no means of curing the disease. Intercurrent infection is a particular hazard which can precipitate intravascular sickling. If prophylactic or early treatment is given to prevent severe infections from developing, much ill health is avoided. When pregnancy occurs in a person with sickle-cell anaemia a dangerous situation arises which is discussed below. In areas where malaria is endemic, children with sickle-cell anaemia should have constant antimalarial prophylaxis, for although the presence of haemoglobin S in the red blood cells of those with the sickle-cell trait reduces the severity of falciparum malaria, it does not altogether prevent it and the stress of even a mild infection may be disastrous .for the patient with sickle-cell anaemia. An adequate diet should be supplemented with folic acid 5 mg. daily.

Attacks of bone pain should be treated with analgesics, such as calcium acetylsalicylate, 1 g. four-hourly or, if necessary, pethidine. The use of drugs that are addictive should be avoided, if possible, since the repeated need for analgesics can be predicted. Dehydration, due to the inability of the kidney to concentrate the urine, must be avoided. A rapid intra-venous infusion of sterile isotonic saline (10 ml./kg. body weight) may dramatically reduce pain in which case this infusion may be repeated every 12 hours for a total of 48 hours, unless there is complete relief sooner. If osteomyelitis is suspected a blood culture will help to identify the responsible organism, which is usually one of the *Salmonella* group. Hence either tetracycline, if the organism is sensitive to it, or chloram-phenicol should be given immediately and continued for at least three weeks and until all signs of infection have resolved.

Blood transfusion is of temporary benefit only and should be reserved for periods of particular risk, such as a fall in haemoglobin below 4 g. per 100 ml. or a severe infection. Transfusion itself is not without risk as the incidence of painful crises is related to increased blood viscosity, which is dependent on the red cell count and the oxygen tension as well as on the amount of sickle-cell haemoglobin in each red cell. Haemolytic crises have also been seen to follow transfusion of compatible blood. Trans-fusion adds to the accumulation of iron which may in later life result in increased hazards due to siderosis. This danger may be reduced by chelating agents (p. **1108**). Furthermore the high incidence of viral in-fections in the tropics increases the risk of serum-transmitted hepatitis. When transfusion is considered necessary only blood of normal haemo-globin type should be given.

Surgery is a particular hazard in sickle-cell anaemia. If even temporary and local anoxia or venous congestion occurs intravascular sickling is very likely. For this reason emergency operations should be avoided whenever possible and tourniquets must never be used. If operation is essential it should be carefully planned so that adequate and continuous oxygenation is assured and the blood pressure and limb temperature maintained at normal levels. In a severely ill patient exchange transfusion with blood of normal haemoglobin type is advisable. The immediate post-operative care should include frequent haemoglobin determinations and blood transfusion should be given if a sudden drop occurs.

Splenectomy is of value only in the very rare instance of a superadded hypersplenism.

Prognosis. It is probable that in Africa, without medical attention, few children with sickle-cell anaemia survive to adult life. With full medical facilities many cases survive as a result of the treatment described above and, although subject to ill-health, lead a satisfying life.

Other Sickle-cell Diseases

The degree of anaemia and the frequency of crises depends upon the stability of the particular combination of haemoglobin within individual red cells. Some haemoglobins, e.g. haemoglobin D$_{PUNJAB}$ and haemoglobin C, react strongly with sickle-cell haemoglobin and crises occur frequently in persons who inherit one of these haemoglobins with sickle-cell haemoglobin. Foetal haemoglobin seems to stabilise sickle-cell haemoglobin. Thus persons who inherit the gene for persistence of foetal haemoglobin as well as sickle-cell haemoglobin may have no clinical disability because although each red cell contains 75 per cent. haemoglobin S it also contains 25 per cent. of the stabilising foetal haemoglobin. When an individual inherits the gene for β-thalassaemia as well as the gene for sickle-cell haemoglobin the result is haemoglobin-S-thalassaemia. This usually causes only moderate anaemia and mild, infrequent crises. In some cases, however, the combination of sickle-cell haemoglobin and thalassaemia traits results in crises as severe as in sickle-cell anaemia and these patients are a considerable anaesthetic risk. Sickling crises arise because some cells contain insufficient foetal haemoglobin to prevent intravascular sickling.

Haemoglobin C occurs almost exclusively in West Africans and their descendants. Because haemoglobin SC disease causes less disability than homozygous sickle-cell anaemia, most patients survive into adult life. Pregnancy seems to be a particular hazard, and in this disease aseptic necrosis of the femoral head, retinal thrombosis causing sudden deterioration in vision and painless haematuria are not uncommon complications. The treatment is the same as for sickle-cell anaemia.

Pregnancy and Sickle-cell Disease

Both sickle-cell anaemia and haemoglobin SC disease carry a high morbidity and mortality during pregnancy. There are three complications which should be particularly noted. Firstly, the occurrence of pregnancy in a person with a chronic haemolytic anaemia results in an additional demand for folic acid and megaloblastic anaemia is usual. Secondly, bone pain crises become much more frequent during the third trimester and particularly during labour and the first two days after parturition. These crises are associated with a high incidence of pulmonary embolism with particles of infarcted bone marrow and sudden death may occur. Thirdly, episodes of sequestration crisis producing severe anaemia with rapid enlargement of the spleen and liver are also a feature towards the end of pregnancy and in the puerperium.

F

These patients need very careful antenatal and postnatal care. They must be given folic acid (5 mg. daily) throughout pregnancy. Arrangements should be made for delivery in hospital and for the patient to live sufficiently close for early admission should a crisis develop during the last trimester. During a bone pain crisis very careful and frequent clinical examination and haemoglobin determination should be made. Exchange blood transfusion may be necessary if there is a sudden fall in haemoglobin either before delivery or in the puerperium. If there is any suggestion of pulmonary infarction, intravenous heparin, in sufficient doses to keep the prothrombin time twice that of normal, should be given and continued until four days after the cessation of symptoms.

Sickle-cell Trait

This is generally a harmless condition but in conditions resulting in abnormally lowered oxygen tension of the blood, intravascular sickling can occur in a person with the sickle-cell trait and the clinical picture of a sickle-cell crisis results. These conditions are encountered at altitudes above 15,000 feet, and thus in high flying in unpressurised aircraft. Another potential hazard is anaesthesia with severe anoxia. Bloodless field surgery can be disastrous.

Even in the absence of a generalised reduced oxygen tension it is claimed that persons with the sickle-cell trait are liable to attacks of haematuria due to infarction of renal papillae and also that they are more likely to develop osteomyelitis due to the *Salmonella* group of organisms than are persons with normal haemoglobin. Nevertheless, as has been mentioned above, there is good evidence that persons with the sickle-cell trait have an advantage over those with normal haemoglobin in that they are less likely to die from falciparum malaria.

Diagnosis. The finding of a positive sickling test in association with a normal appearance of the blood film is presumptive of the sickle-cell trait. The diagnosis can be confirmed by electrophoresis of a haemolysate.

Other Abnormal Haemoglobin Diseases

The other abnormal haemoglobins are less important, but both haemoglobin C and haemoglobin E, when inherited in the homozygous state, result in a mild degree of haemolytic anaemia. In others, although haemolysis occurs, it is adequately compensated for by increased erythropoiesis. The mechanism underlying the haemolysis is not yet clear. Haemoglobin D$_{PUNJAB}$ and haemoglobin E are of special importance if inherited together with β-thalassaemia. The result is a haemolytic anaemia with laboratory and clinical features intermediate in severity between those of thalassaemia major and minor.

THALASSAEMIA

Thalassaemia is an inherited disorder of haemoglobin synthesis, in which there is partial or complete failure to synthesise the polypeptide chains of the haemoglobin molecule. The exact nature of the defect is not yet understood. Beta chain synthesis is most commonly affected. When the abnormality is inherited from one parent only (heterozygote) synthesis of haemoglobin is only mildly affected and little disability occurs. When the patient is homozygous synthesis is grossly impaired and severe anaemia results.

Failure to synthesise beta (β) chains (β-thalassaemia) is the commonest type and is seen in highest frequency in the peoples of the Mediterranean littoral. Heterozygotes have what has been called thalassaemia minor, a condition in which there is usually mild anaemia and little or no clinical disability. Homozygotes (thalassaemia major) are unable to synthesise haemoglobin A and, after the neonatal period, have a profound hypochromic anaemia associated with much evidence of red cell dysplasia and increased red cell destruction. In these patients there is no inhibition of delta (δ) chain production and this is optimally used to give relatively high levels of haemoglobin A_2 ($\alpha_2\delta_2$) (p. 146). Haemoglobin F ($\alpha_2\gamma_2$) production is switched off in the neonatal period, but because of the severe anaemia some production persists and HbF may provide much of the circulating haemoglobin. Thus these patients attempt to supply their requirements with haemoglobins that normally comprise only 3 per cent. of the total. At best they usually manage little more than 30 to 50 per cent. of the normal adult complement of haemoglobin.

The anaemia is crippling and the possibility of survival for more than a few years without transfusion is poor. Bone marrow hyperplasia early in life may produce head bossing, prominent malar eminences and other changes giving a mongoloid appearance. The skull X-ray shows a 'hair on end' appearance and general widening of medullary spaces which may interfere with the development of the paranasal sinuses. Development and growth is retarded and folic acid deficiency may occur. Splenomegaly is an early and prominent feature. Hepatomegaly is slower to develop but may become massive especially if splenectomy is undertaken. Transfusion therapy inevitably gives rise to haemosiderosis. . Cardiac enlargement is common and cardiac failure in which siderosis may play a part is a frequent terminal event.

Diagnosis. Thalassaemia minor is often detected only when iron therapy for a mild hypochromic anaemia fails. The demonstration of microcytes, increased resistance of red cells to osmotic lysis and a raised haemoglobin A_2 fraction together with evidence of the same abnormalities in other members of the family establishes the diagnosis. In contrast haemoglobin A_2 levels are diminished in iron deficiency states.

The diagnosis of thalassaemia major is made by the finding of profound hypochromic anaemia associated with evidence of severe red cell dysplasia, erythroblastosis, and the absence or gross reduction of the amount of haemoglobin A, raised levels of haemoglobin A_2 and haemoglobin F and evidence that both parents have thalassaemia minor.

It is not within the scope of this book to detail the great variation in the severity of the clinical manifestations of thalassaemia that present a spectrum of disease severity rather than two syndromes. It is clear that there are several types of β-thalassaemia but for further study the reader is referred to publications dealing with this subject in greater detail.

Treatment. Transfusion is the mainstay in the treatment of homozygous β-thalassaemia. Nevertheless, it is important to realise that transfusions are not required unless the haemoglobin falls significantly below 7 g./ 100 ml., unless a definite commitment to a transfusion life is undertaken, in which case the haemoglobin level should be maintained between 10 and 12 g./100 ml. At this level the benefit from transfusion is optimal and the transfusion requirements minimal. The intraperitoneal route may be used in the young to conserve veins. Iron therapy is strongly contra-indicated but folic acid supplements are advisable. Attempts to remove iron by the administration of chelating agents may be employed, but at best such therapy fails to keep pace with the iron deposition that results from transfusion therapy (250 mg. of elemental iron in every 500 ml. of whole blood). Splenectomy may be required for mechanical reasons or if it can be shown to be a site of major red cell destruction. Intercurrent infection must be treated vigorously with appropriate antibiotics.

Alpha Thalassaemia. Alpha thalassaemia is found mainly in South-East Asia. There are probably at least two inherited abnormalities, one associated with severe, and the other with mild inhibition of alpha (α) chain production. Heterozygotes of either abnormality are at little disadvantage since α-chain production is adequate. A slight excess of gamma chain production at birth may form tetramers (γ_4), (haemoglobin Bart's) and this can be demonstrated by electrophoretic techniques. The combination of a mild and a severe α-thalassaemia disorder results in a deficiency of α chain production which is short of absolute, so that some normal haemoglobin is formed. There is an excess of beta chains and these form tetramers (β_4), (haemoglobin H) and this may explain the syndrome of haemoglobin H disease. The inheritance of the severe α-thalassaemia abnormality from both parents is incompatible with life and such offspring are stillborn (hydrops foetalis).

Diagnosis. Heterozygotes for α-thalassaemia can be diagnosed with certainty only at birth when a raised level of haemoglobin Bart's is found. This disappears as the production of γ chains is switched off. Thereafter α chain production appears to be adequate and few if any β tetramers (haemoglobin H) form. A mild degree of microcytosis and hypochromia may be present.

Patients with haemoglobin H disease have hypochromic, microcytic anaemia with decreased osmotic fragility and reticulocytosis and classically show multiple inclusions in the red cells when these are incubated with Brilliant Cresyl Blue. In addition haemoglobin H may be demonstrated in a freshly prepared haemolysate by electrophoresis.

The diagnosis of homozygous α-thalassaemia is suggested by the finding of a profound anaemia in a stillborn hydropic baby. Some haemoglobin Bart's may be demonstrable and evidence of heterozygosity in both parents.

Treatment. Most patients with this disorder are asymptomatic. Patients with haemoglobin H disease require management in the same way as patients with β-thalassaemia.

SPLENOMEGALY AND ANAEMIA

A striking feature of medical practice in the tropics is the frequency with which splenic enlargement, sometimes to an extreme degree, is encountered in association with some degree of anaemia. Whereas such presentation in the temperate areas of the world would suggest leukaemia or reticulosis, the more common causes in the tropics are malaria (p. **1119**), visceral leishmaniasis (p. 2), chronic brucellosis (p. **92**), schistosomiasis (p. 72) and cirrhosis of the liver (p. 118).

In some cases it is not possible to attribute the illness to any of these causes, and the terms idiopathic or cryptogenic have been used of the splenomegaly. There is evidence that this splenomegaly is an abnormal reaction to chronic malarial infection. Far from being typical cases of clinical malaria these patients have no fever, and malarial parasites are more difficult to demonstrate in their blood than in the general population. They show evidence, however, of a hyperimmune state; there is a characteristic infiltration of the sinusoids in the liver and bone marrow with mature lymphocytes, and a higher level of malarial antibodies in their serum than in the serum of the general population. It is probably also significant that these patients often respond to long-term malarial prophylaxis and this is the treatment of choice. In many cases the splenomegaly reduces considerably or even disappears altogether. Cessation of therapy results in a reappearance of the disorder, and prophylaxis should be maintained for life. In some cases, splenectomy may appear indicated and considerable improvement in the anaemia and the patient's well-being may accrue. However, it must be borne in mind that splenectomy in such patients may be associated with a greatly increased susceptibility to malarial infection thereafter, if life-long prophylaxis is not included in their treatment.

Accompanying gross splenomegaly, whatever the cause, there is usually anaemia attributable to the haemodilution associated with an enlarged spleen, and this is mainly due to an increase in plasma volume. The reason for this increase is not understood. In addition, some degree of hypersplenism characterised by haemolysis, thrombocytopenia and leucopenia, frequently is present (p. 876).

It should be noted that this idiopathic type of splenomegaly may complicate disorders also associated with splenomegaly. Thus patients with chronic lymphatic leukaemia may present with enormous splenomegaly and this splenomegaly and the associated anaemia may be greatly improved by long-term malarial prophylaxis.

ONYALAI

The name 'onyalai' has been given to a form of thrombocytopenic purpura of unknown origin which occurs sporadically in various parts of Africa. It differs from essential thrombocytopenia in that it affects mainly young male adults, is not prone to relapses and large haemorrhagic bullae on the tongue and buccal mucosa are a conspicuous feature. Haemorrhages from the gastric mucosa, the renal tract and elsewhere may cause death from anaemia. Haemorrhages into the brain may also be fatal. Anaemia should be corrected by blood transfusions and iron medication. In some cases corticosteroids have been reported as being effective in controlling the thrombocytopenia.

N. C. ALLAN

Index

Index

Page numbers in bold type refer to items included in *The Principles and Practice of Medicine*, 10th edition, and which are omitted from this Supplement.

159

Printed by T. & A. CONSTABLE LTD., Edinburgh

Dominica

Venezuela   Guyana
Brazil.

N. South America